WHEN ILL HEALTH
BECOMES YOUR ENEMY

GW01072005

WHEN ILL HEALTH BECOMES YOUR ENEMY

*UNDERSTANDING THE IMPORTANCE OF PSYCHOLOGICAL
FACTORS IN GOOD AND ILL HEALTH*

GILLIAN MOORE-GROARKE
SYLVIA THOMPSON

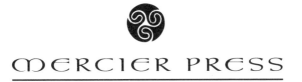

MERCIER PRESS

MERCIER PRESS
PO Box 5, 5 French Church Street, Cork
and
16 Hume Street, Dublin

© Gillian Moore-Groarke & Sylvia Thompson, 1996

A CIP is available for this book from the British Library

ISBN 1 85635 152 X

10 9 8 7 6 5 4 3 2 1

DEDICATED TO
JAYNE

ACKNOWLEDGEMENTS
We would like to thank a number of people who helped us with this book: Charlotte McKenna, secretarary to Dr Moore-Groarke who helped with typing the manuscript, Stephanie Lynch, physical therapist and nurse, Geraldine O'Brien, staff nurse Radiotherapy Unit, Cork University Hospital. All the courageous people who have spoken to us honestly and sincerely about their illnesses and finally to our partners in life James and Des, for their love, patience and understanding.

Printed in Ireland by Colour Books Ltd.

CONTENTS

PREFACE

I'm fairly sure that a visit to my general practitioner of fifty years ago would have entailed a lengthy discussion with him about my life situation in general before he would have prescribed treatment for me. In other words he would have seen my problem in the context of the whole of me and this is the basis of the holistic approach to health care which is explored in this book. This way of looking at things as part of the whole to which they belong is not new. Plato, who lived approximately two thousand years ago, claimed that '... the cure of the part should not be attempted without the treatment of the whole'. It seems to me that despite the wonderful achievements of modern medicine, health care has suffered considerably since this approach was more or less abandoned in favour of specialisation which focuses on parts, treating them in isolation. It would not surprise me if, nowadays, I were to be referred by a general practitioner to a fingernail or eyelash specialist!

I see the holistic model of health care, in its broadest sense, encompassing the body, mind, and spiritual dimensions of the human person. It would look at how the person relates with family, friends, society, culture and environment. Mainstream orthodox medical treatment would be part, but only part, of this approach. There is a growing realisation that the medical model alone has been found to be inadequate when dealing with the many complexities of an illness. Many physicians and hospitals are reclaiming the holistic approach in that they offer a range of natural complementary therapies to patients undergoing medical treatment.

This book, in that it deals with, or hints at, much of the detail of a broad holistic approach, expands the scope and context of illness, healing and well-being. The mind/body connection is so well dealt with that one can easily understand how 'the body speaks its mind' or how that sometimes the body doesn't consider it worthwhile fighting for a life that is not fulfilled or happy. The authors acknowledge the uniqueness of each person; that there are many factors involved in the causes and origins of illness; that we do not 'bring on' our own illness – such a judgement would surely add a further burden of guilt – but that we are often victims of circumstances beyond our control and that such circumstances may be detrimental to our well-being; they suggest that symptoms like dreams, may be pointing to a disease at a deeper level and removing such symptoms without exploring their underlying meaning could be a futile exercise. Being 'positive' means being 'real' even if that includes having to acknowledge feelings that may appear to be 'negative'.

I believe that readers will really appreciate the down-to-earth and do-it-yourself aspects of the book. It offers simple and practical suggestions in the area of self-care through creativity, relaxation, communication, fun and laughter, finding meaning in life. It offers back to all of us the overall responsibility for our own well-being and to those who are ill a sense of having a part to play in their own healing. We are presented with solid scientific data side by side with stories of immeasurable life situations. I find myself trusting authors who in their final paragraph urge us with a quotation from 'Desiderata' to 'be gentle' with ourselves.

Maureen Murphy
SLANÚ Cancer Help Centre
Galway

INTRODUCTION

An interest in psychology among the general public is growing with more and more people signing up for night classes and weekend courses in stress management, relaxation training and personal growth. Such patterns of interest have also been noted in bookshops as more people search the shelves for books like this one to help them understand themselves and their health better. Together with this general move towards self-help is a huge growth in complementary or holistic medicine. Both trends represent a desire for more individual control over life and personal input in the treatment of illness.

For the purpose of this book Dr Moore-Groarke carried out a survey looking at the changes in patients coming to her for counselling in the last five years. The results showed that in 1990 only 30% of patients read self-help books while in 1995 this figure had increased to 85%. 20% in 1990 reported that they had tried a form of complementary medicine compared with 43% five years later. The rate of participation in psychology, stress management courses, etc., had increased five times in a five year period (3% in 1990 and 15% in 1995). Perhaps the most interesting figure of all was the difference in the numbers of patients referred by general practitioners which was 20% in 1990 and 95% in 1995.

In the past, complementary therapies were criticised because of the difficulty of carrying out clinical trials to assess their effectiveness. Now, many family doctors and nurses are also taking courses in psychology and complementary medicine thus increasing the awareness and availability of such therapies. To most complementary therapists, the idea of grouping patients together (e.g., those with high blood pressure) and treating them in the same way is unthinkable – simply because the underlying cause for the disease may be different in each individual. Psychologists also treat people on an individual case by case basis – building up a picture of their health through knowledge of their mental and emotional well-being, past and present life situations, family history, work life, relationships, etc.

Psychology is now a complete subject in most medical degree courses and in many parts of the world, counsellors and psychologists are now part of the team involved in general practice. Such trends can also be seen in the growth of medi-centres throughout Ireland.

In this book we look at different aspects of illness placing emphasis on the psychological component. The underlying theme is how taking an active role in the management of health can help people deal with pain and the anxiety surrounding illness more effectively. The individual's involvement is crucial for their return to good health or in coping with long term or chronic conditions. Such assertions are by no means intended to undermine the role of doctors, natural medicine practitioners and psychologists in the treatment of illness. Instead, the purpose is to stress that without the patient's input such treatments can be wholly inadequate.

The psychological health of ill people is sometimes incorrectly seen to be peripheral to their physical illness. Throughout this book, we attempt to show that it is only when keen attention is placed on such emotional and mental well-being can patient and doctor alike address the illness with strength and hope for a full recovery.

In chapter one, we look at the mind/body connections, and how through its history orthodox medicine has separated mind and body. Complementary medicine shows that in separating the two a very valuable link has been broken and many insights lost. Psychology can in many ways act as a bridge between the two approaches.

In chapter two, we examine stress and offer you a chance to identify your sources of stress with the aim of having better coping techniques. In chapter three, we discuss the psychological aspects and importance of pain (for instance sometimes pain can be a crucial signal to rest the body), giving some helpful suggestions of ways in which you can make pain more bearable through relaxation, visualisation and imagery techniques. In chapter four, we look at the influence of personality on illness and the different patterns of physical and mental illness affecting men and women.

In chapter five, we examine the power of placebo drugs in the context of the psychological factors in illness. We also look at the importance of good communication between professional and patient and how such communication can, in fact, improve the patient's chance of recovery. In chapter six, we look at the growth of health psychology as an integral part of treatment of chronic and acute conditions. We also consider how holistic healthcare can help people understand their illness in all its dimensions.

And finally, in chapter seven, we discuss simple ways in which the use of your own personal psychological techniques can help to improve your health and reduce your chances of suffering from one of the chronic illnesses that are so prolific in our society today.

GILLIAN MOORE-GROARKE

SYLVIA THOMPSON

1

BODY AND MIND

The power of the body is in the magic of the mind
ANONYMOUS

Are the body and mind separate entities or part of an intercon-nected system which links mental and physical health? Has orthodox medicine ignored psychological well-being to such an extent that it has inadvertently stimulated the growth of inter-est in complementary medicine? What role has psychology in this new equation?

A quick skim through the disease patterns in the western world over the past 150 years shows a radical shift in the most prominent types of illness. While such infectious diseases as smallpox, cholera and typhus have largely been brought under control by medical advances, disorders like coronary heart disease, cancer and hyper-tension (high blood pressure) have increased dramatical-ly over the same period.

Some researchers believe that health disorders with a large psychological component make up 30% of the com-plaints now seen by general practitioners. Other studies have put the percentage of illness with a psychological factor as high as 90% of all reported complaints.

General health surveys have also found that half the population suffer from at least one psychosomatic symp-tom (headache, gastrointestinal complaints, hyperten-sion) on a regular basis. Traditionally, such problems (when no physical cause can be found) have been treat-ed with scepticism by medical doctors. Rather than blame the medical profession for a lack of understanding, it is however more interesting to look at the origin of such thinking and see how – as we approach the twenty-first century – the emphasis on physical causes as the only relevant cause of illness is no longer appropriate.

Until very recently, the medical profession viewed the body and mind as separate entities. This way of thinking dates back to the seventeenth century French philosopher, René Descartes who believed that the mind and body were two distinct systems, causing and provoking reactions which were completely unrelated. This philosophical position which became known as dualism, influenced medical practice greatly. It was so strong that it prevented acceptance of the fact that psychological and physical conditions were closely related.

THE MIND-BODY ISSUE
Some scientists believed that the mind-body issue could be solved simply by denying that it was an issue. Others believed that since it was unknown how anxiety, depression or stress could cause a migraine attack or heightened blood pressure, it was best to ignore the problem for the time being. Instead, they put all their energies into learning more about the complex biochemical and neurophysiological processes of the body, i.e., how different organs functioned in conjunction with each other to keep the body in working order.

Medicine itself became intensely specialised with technology playing a larger part in the diagnosis and treatment of different conditions. Such an emphasis on the physiological basis of illness not only reduces the individual to 'a set of walking symptoms' but also placed a great stigma on any illness which didn't have a physiological explanation. 'It's all in the head' is a commonly used expression which reduces someone's suffering to some kind of psychological weakness on their part simply because no organic basis can be found for their symptoms.

The body most definitely has a mind of its own. Mind-body medicine makes many doctors extremely uneasy. They feel it is more a concept than a true field of medicine. Doctors until recently tended to trust the chemical choice of treatments. Drugs do not require any new thinking on the patient's part (or the doctor's) to be effective.

The following case history is an example of how someone can be treated inappropriately by not taking their psychological well-being into consideration.

Darren was an only child. His upbringing was overprotective. He went to private schools, was driven to and from wherever he had to be, was given large amounts of pocket money and anything he asked for, he got. Six months prior to sitting his Leaving Certificate he started to develop panic attacks. He was treated by his GP using several drug interventions but still there was no improvement. His GP referred him to a psychiatrist and he was given anti-depressants. He then developed erticaria (itching) all over his body, and consequently was referred to a dermatologist who prescribed skin creams. Again no improvement occurred. He kept going back to his GP presenting with symptoms such as chest and back pains, visual disturbances, headaches, poor taste and smell. His parents were despairing and finally decided on a friend's recommendation to see a psychologist. The psychologist diagnosed Darren as suffering from stress and anxiety. He immediately started on a stress-management treatment programme, combined with homoeopathic medicine and within three weeks his condition showed tremendous improvement. Once Darren learned to deal with his stress and develop his own autonomy, the erticaria went away. Darren needed to be listened to above anything else. His parents also participated in parts of the treatment programme.

Recent surveys in England and the United States have shown that 80% of patients feel their complaint was not satisfactorily dealt with on leaving the doctor's surgery. Patients reported that they did not feel listened to and the language used by the doctors was difficult to understand. Younger patients were however more likely to ask questions than older ones. Older patients have greater difficulty, when removed from their environment, and adapting to a change of routine causes them great stress. Other studies have shown that psychiatric patients improved more while on a waiting list to see a psychiatrist than actually having seen the psychiatrist. The situation is much more complex than exchanging a body doctor for a mind doctor.

PSYCHOSOMATIC ILLNESSES

People with so-called psychosomatic conditions have suffered from this dualistic approach to illness. Although their symptoms are very real, they have no discernable physiological basis. In some cases, this led doctors to believe that such conditions were not as serious and so were not deserving of the same attention that most organic illnesses were receiving. Thankfully this view, has changed over the past ten years. Canadian psychologist, Donald A. Bakal has argued that the term psychosomatic itself is misleading and should be abandoned. He believes that few illnesses, if any, can be narrowed down to emotional or a physical cause in isolation. The majority of illnesses are instead multifactorial in origin, having both psychosocial and physical causes. Despite what professionals such as Donald A. Bakal believe, the term psychosomatic is still widely used.

Holistic practitioners follow a multifactorial approach to illness and believe that good and ill health results from a combination of emotional, physical, mental and even spiritual factors. Individuals who go to such practitioners for help will be asked much more about their work, diet, exercise and relationships than was generally the tradition within orthodox medicine. *However it is always best to go to your doctor first to rule out any possible physical causes of any disease.*

The following case history is an example of what is referred to as a psychosomatic illness. The physical pain felt by the patient is a clear manifestation of a deep-rooted psychological problem, i.e., the loss of his mother:

> Joe is a retired army officer in his 60s. Six months after his mother died of a stroke, Joe suddenly developed a numbness in his left hand and shoulder. All medical investigations showed negative test results, apart from a slight elevation in blood pressure on admission to hospital. Joe was convinced that he had suffered a stroke and continuously questioned the medical personnel about his diagnosis. One junior doctor told Joe that it may have been a slight stroke, but he could not be certain.
>
> Mary, Joe's wife, told us that every time Joe becomes depressed he talks about the numbness in his arm. When this happens, he becomes socially withdrawn and becomes a closet drinker. Joe refuses to talk about his mother's death, and his strong denial of this major event in his life has manifested itself in the physical numbness of his arm. When Joe finally came to see a psychologist he realised the importance of talking to somebody about his bereavement.

There is now a developing trend within orthodox medicine to involve psychologists in the treatment approach to acute and chronic conditions. We will discuss the applications of health psychology in chapter 6 but here it is interesting to look at how such major illnesses as cancer and heart disease, are now widely believed to have some psychological components.

One biographer of the novelist D. H. Lawrence claimed that the writer died of a broken heart, not tuberculosis which he was diagnosed with. Many close relatives of people who die suddenly from acute conditions or having suffered long-term from chronic illnesses will testify that they feel certain aspects of the individual's personality and/or lifestyle contributed to his/her death. There are links between personality and illness and these are discussed in greater detail in chapter 4.

Every practising physician knows that the patient's will to recover plays a vital part in his/her treatment. Dr Chopra, an Indian endocrinologist working in the United States says, 'Wedded as they are to hard medicine, most doctors nonetheless cannot condone the idea that attitude, belief and emotions do play their part'. Hippocrates was quoted as having said 'A patient who is mortally sick might yet recover from belief in the goodness of his physician'.

Cancer patients are often believed to suffer from an inability to express emotions. It is sometimes thought that as children they lacked a close relationship with their parents. Instead of speaking openly about their feelings, they choose to keep them to themselves. Not opening up about feelings sometimes has an effect on the immune system which can lead to cancerous changes. Internalising emotions rather than outwardly expressing them can also lead to depression.

Studies on breast cancer survival rates in the mid 1980s showed that women who displayed strong positive attitudes tended to outlive those with negative attitudes. Another study found that any strong attitudes needed to be expressed. People were encouraged to fight rather than to give up on the disease.

In his book *Grace and Grit*, Ken Wilbur discusses the spirituality and healing in the life and death of his wife Treya. The chapter 'Condemned to meaning' says that cancer is about 30% genetic, 55% environmental (drinking, smoking, dietary fat, fibre, toxins, sunlight, electromagnetic radiation, etc.) and about 15% emotional, mental, existential and spiritual.

Although, such theories are difficult to prove they do illustrate the extent to which psychological factors are now considered to have a role in the course of curing illness. There is also evidence to suggest that people with certain personality types tend to live longer than others even when they get cancer.

Another condition which many people have come to believe to be influenced by personality is heart disease. People with what has been described as type A personality (i.e., ambitious, aggressive and with an exaggerated sense of time passing) are twice as likely to have a heart attack as more placid, easy-going Type B personalities. In one study, Californian psychologists successfully used Stress Management counselling to reduce Type A traits in men who already had one heart attack. The results showed that the rate of second attacks was significantly reduced, as compared with heart attack victims who had not had counselling.

However, in reality, most people have some Type A and some Type B characteristics. What is now seen to be more significant is a tolerance for stress which varies widely with certain individuals stating that they thrive on it. We will look more closely at personality factors and their relationship to good and ill health in chapter 4.

Louise L. Hay the metaphysical therapist, believes we create every so-called 'illness' in our body. The main criticism of her theories is that she seems to ignore physical or genetic causes of disease, poor nutrition, sociological factors, stress and tension. She sees the body as a mirror of our inner thoughts and beliefs. She believes that between 90%–95% of all illnesses are caused by mental/emotional factors. She takes a variety of illnesses and relates them to unresolved emotional issues. Although, perhaps, oversimplistic and inadequate as the sole cause of illness, it is interesting to consider her theories.

Here are a few examples:

(a) Laryngitis, she says represents the fact that you are so angry you cannot speak.
(b) Tonsillitis and thyroid problems represent problems you have as a result of frustrated creativity, at not being able to do what you want.
(c) Pre-menstrual Syndrome (PMS) she sees this as based on an incorrect concept that the body is dirty.
(d) Anorexia and Bulimia Nervosa she sees as an extreme form of self-hatred.
(e) Arthritis comes from constant criticism and a perfectionist personality.
(f) Asthma she associates with a feeling of being smothered, i.e., you do not even have a right to breathe.
(g) Cancer she sees as an extreme form of resentment.
(h) Obesity indicates an emotional need for protection.

(i) Tumours are a result of unresolved hurts.

Her philosophy and the road to healing involves nurturing and nourishing – the body, mind and spirit. She says if any of these areas are ignored, we are incomplete and we lack wholeness.

We nurture the body with proper nutrition and exercise. The mind is cared for by using one or a number of psychological techniques or therapies which promote positive attitudes. The spiritual aspect of our lives can be addressed through using meditation or practising forgiveness, or a combination of mind and body treatments which leave space for private individual growth.

Illness can be viewed as a 'signal button', to direct our lives. As you read on you will see that we can give ourselves numerous healing messages through psychological techniques. The important role of modern medicine is recognised – but remarkable results can also be achieved through body-mind communication.

2

STRESS AND ILLNESS

Illness is in part what the world has done to a victim, but in a larger part it is what the victim has done with his world and with himself
KARL MENNINGER

What exactly is stress and where does it come from? In what illnesses is stress a major factor? What simple psychological techniques can be learned to reduce stress?

Stress first became a buzz word in America in the 1960s when people's lives started to become more compartmentalised, and time a commodity that always seemed to be in short supply. Nowadays, most people's lives are made up of a timetable of activities, some of which never get the space they deserve. Think for a moment how your average day fills out. Although work takes up a big chunk, for many people there are often different tasks demanding attention. Meal times and leisure activities, which usually involve interactions with family, friends and colleagues, are often all too short. Trying to fit everything in is itself a cause of stress for many people, while not having enough to do can be stressful for others.

While everyone has an increased awareness of what being under stress feels like, few really make the effort to re-organise their lives to reduce stress. Later, we will discuss some simple psychological techniques which can be used to cope with stressful situations and in some cases to avoid them in the first place. But, first it is interesting to look at where the stressful reaction originates from in the body.

Some of our difficulty with stress today is due to the body's primitive response system. The human nervous system has existed for millions of years and it is only in a very small portion of this time, that human beings have had to cope with what is sometimes called civilised stress.

The fight or flight response is the body's natural reaction to stress. Primitive people depended on this physical reaction for survival when confronted by a threat, just like animals continue to do today. The stress response is a defence mechanism which produces effects that permit, in conditions of actual or potential danger, more strenuous effort than normal. The goal is reached by strengthening some mental and physical functions like alertness, heart rate and blood pressure, visual acuity, muscle strength, blood coagulability, pain tolerance and inhibiting some drives like sexual and eating ones that are of no great use in a situation of danger. The problem is that most people nowadays find a fight or flight response to be inappropriate. For example, if you have an argument with your boss, you cannot run away and neither can you physically attack him/her. Instead, you usually have to accommodate what has been said, ignore it or put it aside until later. This 'civilised' reaction makes the physical response redundant, i.e., the nervous system's production of adrenaline to prepare for the fight or flight reaction and the endocrines release of energy into the body for action has no release. It now has to be withdrawn back into the body. It is this lack of release which causes stress and if it occurs regularly leads to ill health.

Stress results when the body fails to utilise the hormones and endocrines brought into action by the fight or flight response. When such a stressful reaction occurs often and over an extended period of time, the physiological arousal systems become over-activated, leaving the body vulnerable. Illness occurs when certain other bodily organs attempt to adapt to this state and in so doing function maladaptively themselves.

A simple example of the above process is found by looking at the action of the heart during the fight or flight response. When the body is under stress, the blood pressure and heart rate both increase. If such an unnatural state becomes a regular occurrence, this puts undue pressure on the heart and blood vessels thus weakening their normal functioning. High blood pressure occurs when the stressful situations are frequently responded to by the body. In other words, the individual feels under stress regularly over a time and the body's stress reaction becomes exaggerated and sustained.

Our immune system does not function well when the body is under stress which directly increases our susceptibility to infectious diseases (e.g., colds, flu, shingles, measles, chicken pox, etc.). Even the common cold will take an unusually long period to clear if you are suffering from a lot of stress at the time. Some food-related allergies are also exacerbated during periods of high stress. Diet management plays an important part in the control of migraine headaches. Yet, when under stress, many migraine sufferers forget precautions (such as avoiding dairy products, spicy foods, red wine, etc.) that they should pay close attention to.

As stated earlier, most of us know well what being under stress feels like but few of us learn to deal with it. Here are two examples of how you can take control of the stress levels in your life.

Ray is 35 and a member of middle management in a busy firm. He is responsible for six company reps. His job also involves a lot of travelling and late nights. He usually spends two nights a week away from home. He has had numerous relationships over the years but has been unable to sustain any of them for very long. Work has always taken first place.

Socially he has to push himself very hard, making contacts and entertaining potential clients. Over time he started to put on weight, and began to feel depressed and lethargic. A holiday he took to get away from it all was a disaster as he developed panic reactions and had to fly home. A visit to his GP led to a referral to a psychologist. The psychologist diagnosed him as suffering from burnout, extreme stress, anxiety and a panic disorder.

The prescription for recovery was a few weeks off work to give himself time to learn to relax and reassess his lifestyle and habits. Ray completed a ten week stress management course and showed a significant improvement. During this course he learned deep muscle relaxation which he practised twice daily, listening to a tape before getting up and before going to bed every day. He prioritised what he had to do every day by making lists and keeping a diary. He learned to slow down in every aspect of daily living. He no longer ran to the phone, instead he took his time or pulled in off the road if his car phone rang. He slowed down eating, talking and driving and consequently he felt less rushed and anxious. Each day he took time out, e.g., for a walk, to listen to music or practise his relaxation skills.

Ray still occasionally finds himself hopping back into top gear. He was open with his colleagues and explained his absence from work. They were very supportive and now each week they meet and discuss their own personal difficulties or work related problems. The company proposed to send all its representatives on stress management courses in the future. What they will spend on courses will no doubt save them on their rate of absenteeism.

Kay is 32, with three children aged 5, 3 and 18 months. Her husband John is a 35 year old bank manager. Since John began pursuing his career, they had eight house moves in their seven years of marriage. Kay gave up her job (she also worked in the bank) when their first child was born.

John leaves home every morning at 8a.m. and Kay is lucky if she sees him any night before 10p.m. Because they have moved so much she has no friends or family living close by. She is with the children all day and longs for some adult company. She only gets to see her family every three/four months.

Any socialising they do, albeit rarely, is usually within banking circles which Kay finds boring and tedious. Most weekends John brings work home with him. Each time she tries to approach him with regard to her feelings, he says his hard work is for the family's sake, so that they would all have a better life and this makes Kay feel guilty.

After another house move, Kay started to lose weight and neglect her appearance. The housework was catching up on her. It was only when her parents came to visit for Easter that she broke down and confided in them. John was extremely embarrassed at what had happened and decided to take time to visit with their GP.

The GP diagnosed Kay as suffering from stress and depression, he advised John that he too was treading on dangerous ground, with regard to his own health. Kay's parents took the children for two weeks and gave them time together.

John agreed to get somebody in to help Kay with housework and they both attended counselling for the following six months. They worked on their relationship, communication difficulties, stress levels and Kay's depression.

The life changes for the better were as follows:

- The communication in their relationship improved.
- They both made time for each other and found it easier to relax.

• They did not let problems mount up but spoke about them as they arose.

This case history illustrates the fact that some people unfortunately await a crisis before dealing with their stress.

STRESSFUL LIFE EVENTS

While many people encounter stressful situations in their everyday lives, there are a number of life events which are known to be particularly stressful. Such events were rated in terms of their stress levels by two American psychologists, Holmes and Rahe. As can be seen from the table on the next page, stressful life events are not confined to negative experiences. Such happy occasions as weddings, childbirth and holidays can incur a lot of stress. How stressful an event is ultimately depends on the amount of change involved and how different individuals react to change.

Illness is more likely to occur during or immediately after a highly stressful event. A simple example of the latter is how a number of people become ill while on holidays. When they stop work, the stress disappears, it is only then that the body has time to be ill.

Ken is a builder in his 30s who went bankrupt. Two days after the liquidators moved in, he suffered a nervous breakdown. Until then he seemed to be coping well. While the stress had not to be so great as to make the body ill immediately (during the stressful situation), instead it affected his mind soon after the stress has been 'coped' with.

Dr Holmes followed up the life events chart with a set of guidelines which are useful as a means of self-evaluation and management of stress. They are as follows:

(1) Become familiar with the life events – and the

Rank	Life Event	Mean Value
Family		
1	Death of a Spouse	100
2	Divorce	73
3	Marital Separation	65
4	Death of a close family member	63
5	Getting Married	50
6	Marital reconciliation	45
7	Major change in physical/mental health of family member	44
8	Pregnancy	40
9	Gaining a new family member (birth, adoption, etc.)	39
10	A major change in number of arguments with spouse	35
11	Son or daughter leaving home	29
12	Trouble with your in-laws	29
13	Spouse beginning or stopping work outside the home	26
14	Major change in family get-togethers	15
Personal		
1	Jail term	63
2	Personal injury or illness	53
3	Sexual difficulties	39
4	Death of a close friend	37
5	Outstanding personal achievements	28
6	Beginning or end of education	26
7	Major change in living conditions	25
8	Change of personal habits (e.g., giving up smoking)	24
9	Moving house	20
10	Changing to a new school	20
11	Changing leisure/social activities	19
12	Major change in sleeping habits	16
13	Major change in eating habits	15
14	Going on holiday	13
15	Christmas	12
16	Minor violation of the law	11
Work		
1	Job loss	47
2	Retirement	45
3	Major business readjustment	39
4	Change to different type of work	36
5	Major change in responsibilities at work	29
6	Change in work hours/conditions	20
7	Difficulties with your boss	23
Financial		
1	Major change in financial position	38
2	Taking out a mortgage	31
3	Foreclosure of mortgage or loan	30
4	Taking out a loan	17

Reprinted by permission of the publisher from Holmes and Rahe, 'The Social Readjustment Rating Scale,' *Journal of Psychosomatic Research*, issue 11, Copyright 1967 by Elsevier Science Inc. 1967) amount of change they may require.

(2) With practice, you can learn to recognise when a life event happens.

(3) Think about the meaning of the event for you and try to identify some of the feelings you experience.

(4) Think about the different ways you might best adjust to the event.

(5) Take your time in arriving at decisions.

(6) If possible, anticipate life changes and plan for them well in advance, e.g., changes might occur in income due to retirement, etc.

(7) Pace yourself. This can be done even if you are in a hurry.

(8) Look at the accomplishment of a task as a part of daily living and avoid looking at such an achievement as a 'stopping point'.

(9) Remember, the more changes you have, the more likely you are to get sick and the more you should take care of yourself.

STRESS-RELATED ILLNESSES

It is not unreasonable to suggest that stress is an integral part of an illness. While, it is most commonly deemed to be a causal factor in heart disease, high blood pressure, diabetes, tension headaches, migraine, irritable bowel syndrome, backache, menstrual problems and some cancers, a high stressed lifestyle also encourages some unhealthy coping behaviours such as cigarette smoking, excessive alcohol intake, poor eating habits and drug abuse, all of which take their toll on physical health and emotional well-being.

Some illnesses such as insomnia, eating disorders, such as anorexia, bulimia and obesity, are also a reaction to chronic stress especially when the patient can find no other way of dealing with the stress. Illness itself can also become a stressor if the patient does not learn appropriate coping techniques while suffering from an acute or chronic condition. In our book on eating disorders, *When food becomes your enemy*, we show how the eating disorder acts as a symptom of something much more deep rooted in several patients.

The following case history is an example of how a holistic treatment programme can be more appropriate for some people suffering from a physical illness:

Malcolm is a 24 year old primary school teacher. For the last two years he has not had permanent work and has acted as a substitute teacher in six different schools. Each time Malcolm's period of substitution was coming to an end, his ulcer acted up again. He was lucky to have a good relationship with his GP who was vigilant enough to realise that medication alone was not going to be sufficient to treat his condition.

He was referred to a psychologist who helped him readdress all relevant areas of his life. Within six months he was off all medication, and showed a great improvement. His treatment programme consisted of correct dietary management, relaxation skills and learning to express (rather than keep to himself) the difficulties in not having permanent work.

Learning how to cope with and reduce stress in your life.

Learning new ways of reacting to stressful situations is one of the most healthy ways of coping with or avoiding such chronic conditions as heart disease, high blood pressure, diabetes, tension headaches, migraine, irritable bowel syndrome, backache, menstrual problems and some cancers. Psychological techniques are also healthier ways of coping with stress than smoking, over-eating or taking excessive amounts of alcohol and drugs.

The single most important issue in learning how to cope with and reduce stress in your life is to know when you are under stress. Until you can recognise your own state of stress and what induces it, you can't begin to look at how best to deal with it.

How stressful certain activities and events are depend on the individual's perception of the event. Different people can handle different levels of stress depending on such things as their early experience of stress, their support systems, their individual temperament, their perceived gain from the situation, their goals and ambitions.

Learning to anticipate stressful situations is also useful in that you can then build in stress-relieving activities to follow such periods of high stress. For example, a student who is about to sit her final exams, can make her preparation time more endurable by booking a holiday with some classmates for when the exams are over. Taking time out from study for a short walk is also useful to help relaxation and enhance concentration.

Questions to ask yourself to find out if you are under stress
(A) WELL-BEING SKILLS
1. How well do you value yourself and invest time in yourself? [e.g., Take a walk, practise relaxation, get your hair done.]
2. How good are you at planning and moving towards goals or objectives? [e.g., Make a time-table or plan.]
3. Do you find it difficult to make a commitment? [e.g., Say yes to going out on social occasions.]
4. How good are you at time management and setting

priorities? [e.g., Address your daily chores in order of importance.]

5. Can you pace your lifestyle in a balanced fashion? [e.g., Learn to balance relaxation time with work and family demands.]

(B) INTERACTION SKILLS

1. How good are you at reaching out to others and asking for help? [e.g., Do you go to the doctor as soon as you start to feel ill rather than waiting for the illness to manifest itself completely?]

2. How good are your listening skills? [e.g., Do you find it difficult to concentrate when given instructions?]

3. Can you comfortably be assertive and say 'no'? [e.g., Do you get drawn into things you would rather avoid?]

4. Can you stand your ground and not be easily manipulated? [e.g., Do you end up doing things the other person's way rather than your way?]

5. Do you avoid confrontation? [e.g., Do you give in for a quiet life?]

6. How happy are you in your home environment? [e.g., Are you happy to be living at home, do you have your own space?]

(C) PERCEPTION SKILLS

1. Can you be flexible if changing your mind makes life easier for you? [e.g, Can you be spontaneous?]

2. Do you give in too easily? [e.g., Do you give up at any sign of stress?]

3. Can you accept your limits as a person? [e.g., Do you push yourself too hard?]

4. Are you still able to use your imagination? [e.g.,

Have you lost your creativity?]
5. Can you engage in positive self-talk rather than negative self-talk? [e.g., Can you reaffirm yourself
and say well-done?]

(D) SELF MANAGEMENT SKILLS
1. Are you exercising your body? [e.g., Are you sedentary
or do you engage in regular exercise?]
2. Are you eating a well-balanced diet? [e.g., Do you eat
at regular intervals, avoid skipping a meal?]
3. Are you gentle with yourself? [e.g., Do you know
when to stop?]
4. Do you find time to relax and let go of tension? [e.g.,
Do you have a hobby you pursue regularly?]
5. Are you learning be less anxious and loosen up? [e.g.,
Can you relax when out socially?]

In order to protect our health, we can regularly clear
away the results of the body's reaction to stress with
appropriate exercise and relaxation. Time to talk things
through after a stressful event is also very useful in that
it allows the mind to clear itself of the complexities
which have arisen in particular situations. Here, we
explain some of the best known, tried and trusted, reme-
dies to cope with and reduce stress in your lives.

RELAXATION
Relaxation is often confused with leisure activities which
are far from relaxing.

Although exercise (dealt with in the following section) is essential for good health, competitive sports can
in fact induce a stressful reaction. Doing nothing at all
can, for other people, be intensely stressful.

Relaxation in its purest form is much more than sitting with your feet up in front of the television. Although this can be a winding down exercise, it is more recreational than relaxing. Real relaxation involves techniques which focus on the body in combination with deep breathing exercises. There are many audio tapes now available which can be used to learn relaxation techniques. Practices such as Yoga, T'ai Chi and Aikedo also include a relaxation component which can then be practised at home.

Relaxation techniques once learned and practised regularly, can give you a greater sense of control over your health and general well-being. It is believed that a levelling out of the body's fight or flight reaction occurs when we put ourselves into a state of rest. Becoming aware of, and then letting go, different parts of the body is crucial to deep relaxation.

TIPS ON CREATING THE RIGHT ATMOSPHERE FOR RELAXATION

(1) A warm (but not stuffy) room with low lights and minimum amount of outside noise is the best environment for relaxation.

(2) Gentle background music helps some people to enter into a relaxed state.

(3) Lying flat on a carpeted floor or on a mat is the ideal position for relaxation.

(4) Most relaxation techniques involve becoming aware of and then releasing different parts of your body, often starting from the feet and moving up towards the head.

(5) Some people find oil burners or incense sticks help them to turn their attention inwards.

Here is the text of a relaxation technique you might like to put it on tape and use it to help you relax. [Source: Dr Gillian Moore-Groarke, 1992.]

I want you to sit or lie in a comfortable position in a room free from disruption and close your eyes. Make sure you are warm, use a blanket if you wish. Take a few deep breaths – in and out – slowly, in and out – slowly, in and out – slowly, now relax. Concentrate on a feeling of relaxation – warm – heavy. Allow your thoughts to drift away, free from worry, free from care. Remember you are in total control and you can stop the tape anytime you want. Become aware of your breathing and any tension in your body. Imagine what it would be like if you were free from tension. Create in your mind a pleasant image, perhaps an image of a place where you know you can relax. The one that works best for me is walking along the seashore. It's a warm sunny day and the waves are lapping up and down. Become aware of sounds in this place. Notice how relaxed you are, breathing – in and out – slowly – in and out – slowly – in and out – slowly. Try to forget all the stresses you left behind to take time out and be relaxed. Start with your toes, curl them up – hold – now relax. Notice how warm, heavy and limp they have become. Tense your feet – hold – now relax. Tense your ankles – hold – now relax. Notice how heavy, warm and limp your lower legs have become. Tense your thighs – hold – now relax. You feel your legs becoming lighter. Tense your buttocks by lifting yourself up slightly – hold – (remember be gentle) now relax. Tense your stomach muscles as tight as you can, feeling the stress – hold – now relax. Notice how the tension disappears and how heavy, warm and limp you have become. You are beginning to really relax. You are enjoying this wonderful feeling of relaxation. Clench your fists as tight as you can – hold – now relax – slowly. Tense your wrists and your lower arms, your elbows – now relax. Pull your shoulders up as far as you can, notice the tension – hold – now relax. Watch your breathing – in and out – slowly, in and out – slowly, in and out – slowly. Lift your head back as far as you can – hold – now relax. Lower your head as far as you can in front of you – hold – now relax. Open your mouth as wide as you can. Notice the tension in your jaws – hold – now relax. Curl up your eyebrows as tight as you can – hold – now relax. Notice the wonderful feeling of relaxation created by you all over your face. Rotate your head slowly to the right. Do not strain yourself in any way – relax. Slowly rotate your head to the left. Notice how heavy, warm and limp your body feels. Become aware of the wonderful feeling of relaxation you yourself have created throughout your whole body. Continue to practise your breathing – in – out – slowly, in and out – slowly, in and out – slowly. Sit or lie comfortably for a few minutes and when you are ready open your eyes, notice how alert you are. You no longer feel as tired as before, you feel completely relaxed, free from worries and free from care and ready to face the world again. You know that any time you feel stressed again that you can return to use this tape – any time or anywhere you want. With practice you will learn to control your stress but never hesitate to seek the advice of a professional. I wish you luck.

EXERCISE

Regular exercise has many advantages from the social to the mental and physical. On a physical level, good exercise (swimming and walking are excellent examples) gets the musculature of the body moving, allows air deep into the lungs and gets the heart to beat faster. When practised with other people, it is a useful social outlet and time-out from brain work.

Common sense should play a part in the choice of exercise. While some people do genuinely find group sports exhilarating, some of the more competitive varieties often involves obsessive training sessions and sometimes leave the body open to unnecessary injury. Walking in the countryside, in a forest or by the sea is infinitely preferable to walking in a city where traffic sounds and air pollution is high.

Aerobic exercise is just as important for the body as the more relaxing, muscle-flexing exercises practised in Yoga or Aikedo. Someone who exercises aerobically for 20–30 minutes (increasing his/her heart rate and oxygen intake) goes through a physical process which actually cleanses the body of any hormonal upset due to stress.

Companies are increasingly emphasising physical fitness in their stress management policies. Many big firms, working with specially qualified stress consultants, have already installed in-house fitness schemes and have found that they have been beneficial in reducing absenteeism and staff turnover. When such schemes are in place many employees express greater job satisfaction and a greater ability to cope with job stresses.

For many people, taking exercise and keeping fit can be an even greater pleasure through joining a health club. Membership offers the chance to exercise in a pleasant and sociable ambience. Most clubs offer a wide choice of exercise – gym, aerobics, weight lifting, etc. Some clubs offer a special fitness assessment and personalised programme with specially qualified staff. It is imperative to mention any medical complaints you may have when you are first assessed at the health club. Before signing any membership forms ask to be shown around and discuss any recommended exercise regimes with your family doctor.

Some clubs, with sophisticated hi-tech facilities can seem expensive, but the membership may also seem a small price to pay for taking such positive action to keep harmful stress out of your life.

VENTING YOUR EMOTIONS

There has been a huge growth in understanding in our society of the need to talk about feelings. Bottling up of emotions often causes the body to take on a defensive posture which over time can lead to such ailments as back and shoulder pain. Not finding someone to talk things through with can also mean that you go over things again and again mentally not allowing your mind, and ultimately your body, to relax. The whole physiological experience of stress is thus experienced again and again.

TIPS ON EXPRESSING YOUR EMOTIONS AND AVOIDING STRESS

1. Get to know your own personality. [Discover your personality type. Find out are you more of a Type A (rushed, anxious) or Type B (relaxed, easy going, laid back) personality type.]
2. Learn to identify the various sources of stress in your lifestyle. [Using a diary make a list of (each day for a month including weekends) what causes you stress. Discuss with your doctor or psychologist.]
3. Avoid perfectionism, when it means expecting too much of both yourself and others. [Be realistic as to what you can achieve. Do not put yourself under pressure to complete assignments in too short a space of time. Adopt the same attitude towards other people.]
4. Avoid unnecessary provoking/confrontational situa-

tions. [Always think things through carefully. Don't bottle frustrations up, but talk calmly and respectfully to the other person.]

5. Learn to say 'no' more often, rather than over-committing yourself. [By committing themselves to too many projects at once, many people put themselves under great stress. This is how people become 'burned out'. Avoid saying everything is 'no problem'.]

6. Do not keep all your worries to yourself. [Find somebody you can trust and do not be embarrassed to say that you cannot cope.]

7. Learn the value of positive thinking. [Try to be positive and learn from the experience of illness, otherwise you are more likely to become depressed.]

8. Acquire the habit of sorting out your priorities. [Always put your own needs first, only then can you give your best to other people.]

10. Learn to delegate effectively. [Don't take everything on board yourself, effective delegation means allowing others to share responsibility and get on with the job requested.]

11. Listening is as important as talking in effective communication. [Listening is a powerful learning experience. Always listen to advice before rejecting it.]

12. In situations where it is inappropriate to verbalise your frustrations, write down how you feel about what has or is happening. [Writing is a powerful tool to help you to think clearly. You can always share your writing with somebody you can trust.]

LEARNING COPING STRATEGIES

Effective coping strategies involve being psychologically flexible, learning to use emotion-focused and problem focused strategies appropriately. Having adequate access to coping resources (e.g., a friend/work colleague who you can tell in an emergency), is also crucial when the stressful situation cannot be coped with alone.

Most stress management courses focus on what is called executive/managerial stress, but many of the executive keys to coping that are taught can also apply to everyday living. Stress Management skills can be applied to our personal and home lives effectively and efficiently.

IMPROVING COMMUNICATION SYSTEMS

Communication improves with regular discussion. It is necessary for every couple to take time away from the family home to talk about any difficulties they have in their relationship, with their children or at work.

DELEGATION

Skilful delegation is essential to managing time well. For the smooth functioning of any home/business, delegation is of paramount importance. Each member of the family should play an important part in completing housework – even the children should be given specific jobs.

ACKNOWLEDGEMENT

This basically means giving credit where credit is due. Otherwise people feel worthless and taken for granted. Women who work in the home full-time often complain of being taken for granted and end up when asked their occupation shyly saying I am only a housewife.

VISIBILITY

Making sure you are accessible to your partner, children and work colleagues. Isolating yourself can cause stress to you and others.

LOYALTY

To be loyal to your family, respect confidences. This is one of the best protections against stress.

ASSERTIVENESS

Project yourself as fair and straightforward. Do not sweep things under the carpet. Try to see all sides.

SELF CONTROL

Avoid panicking, relaxation practised regularly helps this. Tension is infectious and reduces output. Think all situations through carefully, before acting.

3

THE COMPLEXITIES OF PAIN

For all the happiness mankind can gain, is not in pleasure but rest from pain.

DRYDEN, *THE INDIAN EMPEROR, IV*

How much of our pain sensation is a learned psychological response or a real signal of physical illness or injury? What influences an individual's reaction to pain? In what ways can we reduce our suffering through self taught psychological pain control techniques?

Pain is the single most common reason why people seek medical attention yet it is the most difficult aspect of any illness to clearly define. We all seek relief from pain at some stage of our lives whether it be from a headache, backache or sprained ankle or from a more complex form of pain such as that experienced in childbirth or with a condition such as osteo-arthritis. Sampson Lipton, the English neurologist, claimed that over half the population suffer from persistent or recurrent pain.

Although it may not always seem so, there are some advantages to feeling pain. Those who have no pain sensation are more prone to injury because they have no signal which deters them from danger. Children learn not to touch dangerous objects from an early age. Unfortunately, this learning experience sometimes results from an accident with a fire, boiling kettle or a sharp knife. The pain sensation is usually strong enough to make them wary of such objects in the future. The pain from an injury also forces us to rest the injured part of the body. If there was no pain sensation, the bone, muscle or ligament would not receive adequate rest time to heal itself. Pain also tells us when we need help. For example, an aching tooth is a signal to go to the dentist.

Pain can be broadly placed in two main categories – a dull continuous ache sometimes characteristic of back pain or a throbbing sporadic jab familiar to most people who have suffered from toothaches.

People's individual descriptions of pain varies despite suffering from the same or similar conditions. The factors that influence pain as we will discuss later in the chapter, also influence patients descriptions and ratings of pain. Sometimes the pain of an injury or disease never completely disappears with healing or other pains appear for no apparent reason, and then recur or never subside.

It is possible to get a more accurate idea of a patient's level of pain through a questionnaire devised especially for this purpose. One of the best classifications of pain sensation, according to the words used to describe pain can be found in the McGill Pain Questionnaire (see table 1 on next page). This questionnaire was devised by Ronald Melzack, a professor of psychology at the McGill University in Canada.

Such a pain questionnaire not only gives the patient a more active role in understanding the pain but it also helps the professional to categorise the intensity of the pain experience therefore aiding decisions on treatment.

As can be seen from the table on the next page there are twenty groups of words. If the words in one or more groups do not fit the pain, the patient does not select any in that group or groups. The words are graded in intensity when totalling the final score. The positions of the

Table 1: McGILL-MELZACK PAIN QUESTIONNAIRE

1 Flickering
  Quivering
  Pulsing
  Throbbing
  Beating
  Pounding
	8 Tingling
	  Itchy
	  Smarting
	  Stinging
		15 Wretched
		  Binding
		  Periodic
		  Constant
		  Brief

2 Jumping
  Flashing
  Shooting
	9 Dull
	  Sore
	  Hurting
	  Aching
	  Heavy
		16 Annoying
		  Troublesome
		  Miserable
		  Intense
		  Unbearable

3 Pricking
  Boring
  Drilling
  Stabbing
  Lacerating
	10 Tender
	  Taut
	  Rasping
	  Splitting
		17 Spreading
		  Radiating
		  Penetrating
		  Piercing

4 Sharp
  Cutting
  Lacerating
	11 Tiring
	  Exhausting
		18 Tight
		  Numb
		  Drawing
		  Squeezing
		  Tearing

5 Pinching
  Pressing
  Gnawing
  Cramping
  Crushing
	12 Sickening
	  Suffocating
		19 Cool
		  Cold
		  Freezing

6 Tugging
  Pulling
  Wrenching
	13 Fearful
	  Frightful
	  Terrifying
		20 Nagging
		  Nauseating
		  Agonising
		  Dreadful
		  Torturing

7 Hot
  Burning
  Scalding
  Searing
	14 Punishing
	  Gruelling
	  Cruel
	  Vicious
	  Killing
		PPI 0 No pain
		1 Mild
		2 Discomforting
		3 Distressing
		4 Horrible
		5 Excruciating

Source: Melzack, R., 1975

words selected are added together – e.g., so many first, seconds, thirds and so on within a group – the lower down within a group the higher the score.

The questionnaire is divided into different sections because different people have different reactions to pain. Groups one to ten are sensory words – what the patient actually feels. Groups eleven to sixteen assess the effect of the pain on the person or what they think about it. Groups seventeen to twenty comprise of the miscellaneous descriptions which do not fit elsewhere.

There is one added feature in the McGill Pain Questionnaire. You will see a section at the bottom of the list labelled PPI (Present Pain Intensity). The patients are asked to fill in their estimate of the level of pain at the moment, on a simple scale of zero to five.

Table 2 on page 46 is an example of a patient's completed questionnaire following a caesarean section.

The simplest method to use to measure pain is the visual analogue scale (see illustration below). This involves giving the person whose pain you want to measure a piece of paper with a line drawn on it, and asking him/her to imagine that the line represents his pain. At one end of the line there is no pain at all, while the other end represents the worst possible pain that the person can ever imagine. In other words, the line is a personal or subjective thermometer of pain. The person is asked to mark on the line a point which he/she thinks measures the amount of pain felt at a particular time. The VAS line is usually 10 cm long. Comparisons can be made on a daily basis.

Visual Analogue Scale

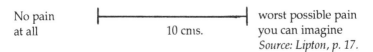

No pain at all — 10 cms. — worst possible pain you can imagine
Source: Lipton, p. 17.

Table 2: McGILL-MELZACK PAIN QUESTIONNAIRE

1 Flickering Quivering Pulsing Throbbing Beating Pounding	8 Tingling Itchy Smarting Stinging √	15 Wretched Binding Periodic √ Constant Brief
2 Jumping Flashing Shooting	9 Dull Sore Hurting Aching √ Heavy	16 Annoying Troublesome Miserable Intense √ Unbearable
3 Pricking Boring Drilling Stabbing Lacerating	10 Tender √ Taut Rasping Splitting	17 Spreading Radiating Penetrating Piercing √
4 Sharp √ Cutting Lacerating	11 Tiring Exhausting √	18 Tight √ Numb Drawing Squeezing Tearing
5 Pinching Pressing √ Gnawing Cramping Crushing	12 Sickening Suffocating	19 Cool Cold Freezing
6 Tugging Pulling Wrenching	13 Fearful Frightful Terrifying	20 Nagging √ Nauseating Agonising Dreadful Torturing
7 Hot Burning Scalding Searing	14 Punishing Gruelling Cruel Vicious Killing	PPI 0 No pain 1 Mild 2 Discomforting √ 3 Distressing 4 Horrible 5 Excruciating

This questionnaire was completed 24 hours post-op by a woman whose baby was delivered by caesarean section and she found it useful in that it helped her explain better how she felt.

Sometimes patients ask themselves what have they done to deserve severe pain. They often think back and make a connection between some action and the onset of pain. Louise Hay bases her theories on this premise but many people believe differently. Pain patients frequently say that they could stand their pain much better if they could only sleep better at night. They believe their resistance is weakened by their lack of sleep. They complain of feeling worn out and exhausted. They become more irritable with family and friends. Their interests wane and they become more self-focused. Sadly, their world begins to centre around home, doctors and hospitals. Chronic pain sufferers (e.g., those with MS, arthritis, severe back pain) sometimes promise to be kinder, to do charity works, if the pain is removed, while others ask for spiritual guidance.

FACTORS INFLUENCING PAIN

How people react to pain depends on a whole host of factors which include individual temperament, family history and cultural values as well as the type of pain itself. Psychological reactions to pain are largely determined by a patient's past experience of pain and the degree of threat and frustration inherent in the pain itself. For example, if someone with a hereditary heart condition develops a chest pain, he may over-react and immediately suspect the worst. In such circumstances, it can be difficult for professionals to convince the patient that his/her chest pain will pass if he/she relaxes.

Some individuals learn from an early age that expressing painful symptoms gives them certain privileges. For example, a phantom tummy ache is a well known child's trick for getting a day off school. Older people sometimes resort to constant complaints of pain as a means of getting extra attention from the people around them. Full-time carers usually come to understand the difference between such attention-seeking and real pain, which needs medical attention.

Physical condition – Psychological reactions to pain are usually greater in weak and tired individuals. The more tired and distraught the person feels, the less tolerant he/she is of pain. The classic example here is a woman's experience of childbirth. The longer the labour, the less tolerant many women become of the pain of childbirth. It is for this reason that many gynaecologists induce the baby's birth after approximately twelve hours of labour. Cancer patients are often tired from long inpatient stays and this also influences their ability to cope with pain. Taking baths, getting adequate sleep (even if this means sometimes taking painkillers prescribed by your doctor to allow you to get asleep) and taking fresh air and exercise (if possible) helps to comfort and relax the body in pain. Being aware of how your body needs to be looked after is sometimes a subtle way of relieving or distracting yourself from pain.

Emotional state – Some people are by nature more emotional about things. Others go through periods of emotional highs and lows at different stages in their lives. Generally speaking, a heightened emotional state exacerbates the pain sensation. For example, a student about to sit his final exams will have a higher level of pain than normal if he has to have his appendix removed before his exams, because of the stress. Sometimes the origin of the pain poses a threat of a more serious illness which worries the patient sufficiently for him/her to feel greater pain. For example, a patient who has been diagnosed as having osteo-arthritis may complain of numbness or loss of feeling in his/her limbs which results in their dropping things. In this instance, the patient's underlying fear of developing multiple sclerosis, can dominate their reaction to pain. Pain sufferers should honestly assess their emotional state to see if they are over-reacting to the pain sensation in any way. Look to see if there are any personal, relationship or other family health problems which are adding to the worry of illness. Such problems may not always be solvable but sometimes becoming aware of their relevance may help to reduce their impact on the physical pain experienced.

Previous pain experience -- Pain responses may be either increased or decreased by the memory of previous pain. Miscarriage, difficult pregnancies or labour often leads to increased stress regarding pain in subsequent pregnancies. People who have suffered from difficult asthma attacks or severe epileptic fits often show great signs of distress during a weaker attack due to their memory of worse experiences. Psychological techniques of relaxation, imagery or music therapy discussed later in this chapter can help to reduce the pain sensation which has been exacerbated due to previous bad experiences.

Perceived significance of pain – When the source of pain is not understood, people sometimes have an exaggerated pain sensation. For example, patients awaiting the results of a biopsy usually show greater pain reactions than those who have just received a negative test result for malignancy. Similarly, many women feel greater soreness from lumps or growths on their breast before they have been diagnosed non-malignant. Some women to whom we spoke when asked to estimate the size of their growth/lump, greatly over-estimated its size while waiting for test results. Once these results came through and were benign, their initial perception disappeared. Fear of the unknown is a common anxiety and can only be truly overcome with information about the illness and reassurance from professionals.

Distraction from pain – When a patient focuses all of his/her attention on the pain, reactions are more pronounced. Because of their distraction from pain, men and women involved in competitive sports are often unaware of an injury until after the game is over. Older people sometimes become so focused on pain that their conversations are limited to talking about how they feel all the time. Their expectation of change following any medical intervention thus becomes far greater and this can lead to disappointment and depression. Learning how to distract oneself from pain is crucial for anyone suffering from a chronic illness. Music therapy, relaxation and imagery techniques are all useful ways of distracting oneself from pain.

The intensity and duration of pain – Intense pain often makes people feel more threatened by their condition. For example women who regularly suffer from severe period pain have a higher pain tolerance than women who rarely have period pains. Pain of long duration such as arthritis is wearisome. Some people resign themselves like martyrs to a life of pain while others take a more active approach, learning to find new ways of tolerating pain. It is useful to look at how you handle pain to see if your behaviour or attitude lowers your pain tolerance in any way.

Personality and family environment – Extroverts are believed to have higher pain thresholds and greater pain tolerance than more reserved and introverted individuals. Those who constantly worry about their health are less tolerant of pain and hypochondriacs have virtually zero pain tolerance. Children who are unhappy are also more likely to grow up with a vulnerability to pain. Emotionally disturbed children sometimes find expression of their problems through painful illnesses. Similarly, individuals who have relationship or marital difficulties can have lower pain thresholds. Such social and psychological factors are rarely given enough attention in the treatment of illness. Throughout this book, our aim is to help people understand how aspects of their lives may contribute to their own pain and how with a better understanding, of their circumstances and lifestyle, they can change certain aspects to improve their condition or at least their ability to tolerate and live with their illness better. This, of course, can only be explored once a you have checked with your doctor that your symptoms are not masking any serious medical problem. For this reason it is imperative that your GP is your first port of call.

Age and sex – As we get older, we are better able to tolerate superficial pain from headaches or period pain and less able to tolerate deeper pain from conditions such as arthritis or chronic back pain. Although men and women are believed to have equal pain thresholds women tend to tolerate pain better for shorter periods of time than men. Finding the most appropriate help for pain relief can be difficult. We will deal with the available options later in the chapter. Below is an example of someone suffering from chronic pain:

Margo, is a woman in her 50s who developed osteo-arthritis six years ago. Margo is a typical Type A personality. She works hard and also cares for her elderly mother who is also arthritic. In a very short space of time the arthritis which began in her hands travelled to her spine and hips. Now six years on, the arthritis has rapidly spread throughout her whole body. Physiotherapy and gold injections have given short-term relief, but the pain is with her every day. She finds herself having to slow down. She drops things easily and each evening her hands and legs noticeably swell.

She also has difficulty sleeping, and often spends most of the night reading. She describes the pain as 'a nagging wearisome pain, which never really goes away'. Her mother became resigned to her pain ten years ago when she was first diagnosed. She now uses a zimmer-frame and suffers from depression on and off, although she will never admit to this.

Margo is determined not to become like her mother. She keeps busy (her husband and children told us that she can never be comfortable for long periods sitting down). If she relaxes for too long her muscles go into spasm. An ulcer prevents her from taking strong analgesics. A neglected whip-lash over thirty years ago seems to have triggered her condition.

Provided she retains the will to keep going her prognosis is as good as anyone can expect. She is one of the few 'silent sufferers'. She uses the coping strategy called 'vigilance' (i.e., facing up to/confronting) which means she faces her pain in a challenging way. She focuses on the positive aspects of her life, and this helps to maintain her endurance.

PAIN INTERVENTION

When left unrelieved, pain leads to physical and mental exhaustion, disablement and chronic anxiety. Eventually some form of medical, psychological and/or alternative intervention becomes necessary. In the following pages, we will summarise the most common approaches used in pain reduction before explaining in more detail the psychological techniques which can help people to tolerate pain more easily and in some cases, reduce the sensation of pain.

1. Drugs intervention

The three main drug types are aspirin containing drugs, opiates and tranquillisers. Aspirin containing drugs reduce inflammation or swelling. Opiates such as morphine, codeine, etc., suppress pain by mirroring or imitating the effect of the body's own natural pain killing hormones. Tranquillisers reduce the mental anxiety which often accompanies physical pain. They help the mind to relax and allow the body to cure itself.

2. Surgery

Surgery is an irreversible form of pain control best approached with the utmost care and as a last resort. Before having surgery, the following questions should be asked of your doctor:

> If I don't have the operation, will my condition deteriorate?
>
> What are the chances of a successful operation?
>
> What are the risks of the operation and what are the risks of the anaesthetic?
>
> Are there any alternative solutions worth trying before deciding on surgery?

3. Acupuncture

Acupuncture is becoming a popular alternative approach to pain relief. It is based on the principles of Chinese medicine which sees the body in terms of energy channels or meridians. When these channels become blocked, the energy flow is impeded which results in pain or illness to the body. An acupuncturist places fine needles at specific points along the meridians to unblock them, thus allowing energy to flow freely again.

4. Hypnotherapy

Hypnosis has been used successfully to increase the pain threshold and tolerance of individuals by helping the patient to focus his/her mind away from the pain. Some people have even undergone surgery (without anaesthetics) under hypnosis. However, not everyone is susceptible or suggestive to hypnosis. The practice of self-hypnosis as a relaxation technique to reduce the experience of pain is something we will deal with later in the chapter.

5. Physiotherapy

Many people with chronic pain are referred to physiotherapists for pain relief. Heat or ice treatment are commonly used in physiotherapy to reduce pain. Ice is generally used in the initial stage to reduce inflammation, etc. Heat is applied in a localised area to bruises, tears, strains or joint inflammation and is used for more chronic conditions such as back pain and joint problems.

6. TENS machine (transcutaneous electric nerve stimulation)

The TENS machine is commonly recommended by physiotherapists but can be used by patients themselves when they know and understand how to use it as a means of inhibiting the passage of pain impulses. It works by stimulating the body to produce its own pain relieving hormones, (endorphins) and has been used by many women during childbirth and by those who suffer from persistent back pain.

PAIN CLINICS AND SPECIALISED CARE

Multi-disciplinary pain clinics have been established in

the United States and Europe. The team of medical specialists at such pain clinics include oncologists, endocrinologists, anaesthetists and orthopaedic specialists, etc. They also include health psychologists, social workers and specially trained nurse therapists. In Ireland people suffering from severe pain or migraine might be referred to the neurological clinic of one of the following hospitals, Cork University Hospital, Limerick Regional Hospital, Adelaide Hospital, Dublin 8, St Vincent's Hospital, Dublin 4 or Galway University Hospital. Some anaesthetists also treat people suffering from chronic pain. 'Slanú' the holistic centre for cancer in Galway teaches many techniques to cope with pain and chemotherapy.

Palliative medicine plays an important role in patient care and the management of pain. This branch of medicine sets out to relieve patients suffering from terminal illness. It acknowledges that pain and suffering can be physical, psychological, social and spiritual. It also involves the patient's family. Most people think of palliative medicine as only applying to cancer patients but now its applications include the care of Aids sufferers and hospice care.

The growth of sports medicine/injury clinics throughout Ireland is also based on the multi-disciplinary approach adopted by such pain clinics and specialised care programmes. Most sport injury clinics now have medical personnel working with physiotherapists and practitioners of complementary therapies.

PSYCHOLOGICAL INTERVENTION IN CONQUERING PAIN
Used in conjunction with other approaches, psychological techniques will not necessarily eliminate pain but can most certainly reduce it. By improving the sufferer's overall quality of life, psychological techniques can also

reduce the patient's dependence on drugs.

Traditionally, the psychologist was only seen as having a role to play in addressing psychiatric illnesses. However, in the last ten years, more and more GPs are referring patients with serious illnesses or those recovering from severe accidents to psychologists for help in dealing with the emotional readjustments and changed life conditions following ill health. The following are some of the areas a psychologist would address in such circumstances.

Confront your pain
Many patients take a passive attitude and role to their pain. However, upon diagnosis (and even before) of a specific condition, it is important that the patient takes an active role in his/her treatment. Building up a support network of family and friends is helpful. Discussing with your boss how best to reorganise your work so as not to exacerbate your pain is also a positive step. Acting the martyr is just about the worst approach to take.

Control your stress levels
Examining your lifestyle and then reorganising your schedule to reduce stress is a very useful task. Stress management courses are helpful for those who can't find the time to organise their own time. Prioritising daily activities and learning not to expect too much of yourself is essential to anyone suffering from chronic pain.

Relaxation
Relaxation techniques such as deep breathing are very effective in reducing the frequency and severity of pain from migraine, backache, arthritis, cancer, labour pains, etc. Taking time out to practise such techniques helps

patients to feel refreshed and ready to face the day or when used at night, they help induce a relaxed and deep sleep. Gentle yoga exercises can also be helpful in strengthening the body during some illnesses.

Hypnosis
Once a clinician determines a patient's suggestibility to hypnosis, the patient can then learn the technique of self-hypnosis. This is most often achieved by producing a tape to induce the hypnotic state for the patient. Hypnosis is seen to be useful in treating pain conditions associated with burns, cancer, migraine, obstretics, dental extractions and surgery. Self-hypnosis reduces pain by modifying the emotional response to pain (i.e., teaching the individual to relax in the presence of pain).

Music therapy
The Indians were the first to recognise the relaxing effects of listening to music. Apart from its soothing qualities, music also works as a good distraction from pain. For example, if you have a back problem and have to drive a long distance, pleasant music can help you to turn your mind away from any discomfort. In many theatres throughout hospitals, some anaesthetists play music to relax the patients scheduled for surgery. Currently, research being done at the Royal Marsden hospital in London shows patients who have their favourite music played while undergoing surgery, or in after care, recover more quickly.

Imagery techniques
The use of images helps to retrain the mind to focus on positive rather than negative attitudes towards pain. For example, someone suffering from cancer can be encour-

aged to think of his/her immune system as a strong powerful army attacking the cancer rather than as a wilting or withering flower unable to exist. Others prefer more tranquil images, e.g., their pain being swept along on the crest of a wave or sinking in the sand. Such images help to build up a better sense of well-being. Also, setting goals to create a more positive attitude, such as someone suffering from back pain saying 'I will ride a horse again' instead of believing that they never will, leads to a more positive attitude. But remember being positive also means being realistic.

TEN POINT PLAN FOR CONTROL OF PAIN

1. Know your illness – try to find out all you can. Talk to other sufferers and do not be afraid to talk openly to your doctor about your fears.
2. Use drugs wisely – only take drugs that have been prescribed for you personally. Never take more than the recommended dosage without prior consultation with your doctor.
3. Use your imagination – try to learn some imagery techniques to focus your attention away from the pain.
4. Learn to laugh – laughter is often described as the best medicine. Watch a good comedy on video or go to an entertaining show. Avoid moaners and negative thinkers.
5. Sleep – get sufficient sleep. If you have difficulty sleeping try to learn to cat-nap or rest during the day.
6. Avoid resignation. Do not just resign yourself to a life of pain.
7. Be assertive – improve your self-esteem. Do not let yourself pay less attention to your appearance as

this will make you look and feel miserable. Always pay attention to personal hygiene.
8. Rest – learn when and how to rest. Listen to your body, if pain increases or returns, remember this is your body's way of telling you it does not like what you are doing.
9. Massage – consider having a massage which will help you to relax as well as loosening up painful muscles.
10. Join a support group – meeting other people who are experiencing the same pain as you helps overcome the isolation that many ill people feel. Remember, pain is not purely physical, it also has important psychological and social aspects.

The use of psychological techniques within the treatment approach of specific conditions

Arthritis

Few diseases affect as many people as arthritis and few cause as much pain and disablement. It is estimated that as many as one in five people will suffer from some form of arthritis in later life.

The standard treatment for arthritis involves drugs. However, the TENS machine mentioned earlier has shown to be more effective than paracetamol in some cases. While it is important to keep reasonably busy and exercise when possible (walking or swimming are good forms of exercise) it is imperative to rest when the pain is severe. Relaxation, maintaining the correct body weight, eating appropriately and significantly reducing stress will all enhance the overall quality of lifestyle for the arthritic patient.

Backache

Between a quarter and a third of the population suffer from backache. In the majority of cases, there are no apparent physical abnormalities and only about 10% of sufferers consult a doctor – but everyone should have it checked by a doctor to make certain the pain is not masking a serious medical condition. Stress and worry are often contributing factors.

Backache can best be controlled by rest when the pain is at its worst. Correct posture must be learned and practised as a life-long skill and not just for the duration of the pain. The Alexander technique is a postural approach which embraces all aspects of an individual's lifestyle in its attempt to alleviate back pain. Yoga also helps to improve poor posture.

Maintaining correct body weight according to the medical mass index with regular exercise also helps. Some sufferers have shown a sustained improvement from regular massage, heat and ice treatment, sitting in a comfortable chair whenever possible, the TENS machine and regular use of relaxation techniques.

Cancer

Approximately one-third of cancer patients suffer some pain. The Simontons who work in the United States highlighted the successful use of imagery techniques as a useful psychological intervention in the treatment of cancers. Attitudes regarding self-confidence and assertiveness are very important for the cancer patient as treatment progresses. Patients also need to be sensitively informed about any changes or deterioration in physical appearance that will occur as a result of chemotherapy.

Headaches

Four out of five people suffer from headaches. Many

people who suffer from frequent headaches fear brain tumours and this, as we explained earlier, can increase the occurrence or severity of the headache. Headaches are in fact often caused by mental tension or emotional stress – but everyone should be checked by a doctor to make certain the pain is not masking a serious medical condition, e.g., tumour, epilepsy, etc.

Relaxation techniques work well in reducing the frequency and severity of headaches. Imagery techniques have also been useful in distracting focus away from the pain.

4

PERSONALITY AND ILLNESS

Your health is bound to be affected if day after day, you say the opposite to what you feel, if you grovel before what you dislike and rejoice at what brings you nothing but misfortune.

BORIS PASTERNAK IN *DR ZHIVAGO.*

Are certain people more prone to illness than others? Is there a valid link between Type A personality profile and heart disease? Are emotionally withdrawn people more likely to develop cancer? Are personality patterns linked to such conditions as migraine, rheumatoid arthritis, etc.? Why do men and women suffer from different mental and physical illness patterns?

Just as you can, to a certain extent, choose what your world will be for you so too can you address destructive personality traits. Awareness of such traits is important in encouraging us to examine our attitudes and psychological orientation, so that in turn we can take many positive preventative steps and measures.

Linking personality types and characteristics to certain patterns of illness is something that has interested psychologists as far back as Freud. Just as certain people cope less well, when they are sick, it is believed that some personalities types are more prone to illness than others. For example, sufferers of asthma, migraine and high blood pressure have often been thought to show distinct personality traits which in some way explains why they developed the condition to begin with.

Individuals with poor coping skills have also been found to have greater immune disruption and to develop a greater number of illnesses than those with good coping skills. The American psychologist Stanley Kobasa identified and measured a style of coping called 'Psychological Hardiness' within which he defined three main components linked to illness. Those who scored high on commitment, control and challenge within the psychological hardiness coping scale were found to be less susceptible to illness.

Although it may sound like a Victorian notion, a hardy family attitude to health has also been found to help those who do face chronic or acute illness. Each individual's attitude to good and ill health is highly influenced by their familial environment. Someone who grows up with a parent who constantly suffers from ill health is much more likely to be a hypochondriac than someone whose parents enjoy excellent health.

The family's attitude and reaction to health and sickness is a subtle determinant of the individual's later approach to illness. Such things as the importance of healthy eating and regular exercises are not always strong features of healthy families yet those who do accommodate the above in their everyday lives are often less prone to infection and illness.

In medicine, it is often disputed whether personality types can be linked to the causation of organic disease. In order to make a link between the physiological and psychological mechanisms, the two must be observed for several years. Many doctors and psychologists consider personality or behaviour traits to be critical in the chain of events. The level of stress combined with the life events an individual experiences are important determinants of how such stress is likely to show itself.

Sigmund Freud believed that physical disorders occur when an individual cannot find an acceptable way to discharge his/her emotional impulses. For example since a strong hostile emotion is generally inappropriate or unacceptable to express, the person unconsciously hides it. This is a learned behaviour since childhood. In such a way, the hostile behaviour is not expressed because the impulse is repressed or inhibited. However, such a mental process can result in the body finding another way of discharging the impulse through physical illness, e.g., colds, flu, headaches, etc.

Following from this analysis, Freud and his followers believed that many physical conditions such as migraine, hypertension, etc., have gone underground or become unconscious. Unconscious feelings of hostility were believed to be one of the triggers of cardiovascular disorders such as migraine and hypertension, whereas unconscious feelings of dependency or desire to be loved were believed to trigger gastrointestinal and respiratory disorders, asthma, etc.

Ulcer patients according to psychoanalytical theories were thought to suffer because they wished to be loved and cared for like a child. Such a wish was repressed because if it was part of the individual's conscious reality, they would experience guilt and shame for having such an infantile need. To avoid awareness of either of the above processes, ulcer patients are said to develop defensive characteristics of pseudo independence and driving ambition. Such compensatory traits did not however prevent the body from having a physiological state of need which resulted in an ulcer. However recent research puts forward the theory that ulcers are a result of a bacterial infection and treatment procedures based on this premise are in the experimental stage.

Further psychoanalytic studies went on to link conditions such as eczema with repressed exhibitionism (i.e. showing the body in order to obtain attention, love and favour) and rheumatoid arthritis with a repression of rebellious tendencies.

Richard Totman in *Mind, Stress and Health*, discusses two American psychologists Grace and Graham who, in the 1950s, argued that an individual's perception of the world, and what s/he thinks about threat, predicts what psychosomatic disorder will develop. They interviewed 128 patients with a variety of diseases to find out what situations immediately preceded the onset of the symptoms and how the individual perceived what was happening to him/her.

They found specific thoughts associated with specific illnesses. For example, individuals with high blood pressure were in a state of constant preparation to meet all threats, and when confronted with threat they thought 'Nobody is going to beat me, I'm ready for anything'. The table below lists other illnesses and the associated thought processes.

ILLNESS	COGNITION/THOUGHT
1. Hives	Perception of mistreatment
2. Eczema	Being prevented from doing something and helpless to deal with the frustration
3. Asthma	Wishing the situation would go away or someone else would take over the responsibility for it
4. Diarrhoea	Wishing to be done with the situation and have it over with
5. Constipation	Grim determination to carry on even when faced with an unsolvable problem

6. Ulcer	Revenge seeking
7. Migraine headache	Engaged in an intense effort to carry out a definite plan

Such theorising is by its very nature flawed because of the difficulty in validating specified emotions/thoughts in their repressed or unconscious form (also because not all people with the given emotion/thought will suffer from the specific condition, and not all patients with the particular condition showed the predetermined characteristics – repressed or otherwise). It is still, however, interesting to consider the study of personality characteristics alongside other causes, and their influence on illness continues to be a subject of interest for both lay people and professionals.

PERSONALITY PATTERNS AND HEART DISEASE

The following is a case history of someone who examined his lifestyle after a heart attack:

> Eamon is in his 50s. Eighteen months ago he suffered a heart attack. He works as a contractor. His wife Isabel says that Eamon is a very stressed person and she notices that he always becomes irritable when he doesn't see much work in sight. Eamon has a typical Type A personality. He works very long hours and is a constant worrier. In the week prior to his heart attack, Isabel said she had noticed that Eamon was very restless. Since the heart attack, he now takes aspirin on alternative days. He was encouraged to give up smoking, practice relaxation and go for a short walk every day. Although luckily, Eamon is not overweight, apart from his work he is virtually sedentary. He had no interest outside his work and his wife is at his constant beck and call. When he was at home the cardiologist encouraged Eamon to attend a 6 week rehabilitation pro-

gramme which examined the quality of his lifestyle. He is now much more relaxed and even his employees have commented on how much more pleasant and amicable Eamon has become.

One of the conditions which has received the most attention on the personality/illness debate is heart disease. While the major physical factors in heart disease such as a high cholesterol diet, elevated blood pressure and cigarette smoking are well documented, it is seldom pointed out that these physical factors are absent in nearly 50% of all new cases of coronary heart disease. This fact has been supported by the American and the Irish Heart Foundations.

In the 1970s, two American cardiologists, Friedman and Rosenman first highlighted the links between certain personality traits and a predisposition to heart disease. They believed that there was a specified behaviour pattern, called coronary-prone behaviour or Type A behaviour which may contribute more to heart disease than all the physical risk factors combined.

The Type A individual was described as being very competitive, aggressive, impatient, restless, hyper alert, explosive in speech, tense in facial musculature and constantly under pressure of time and work responsibilities. Such a personality was thought to have been part of a coping style geared towards asserting and maintaining control over potentially uncontrollable situations.

Studies showed that when Type A individuals – who had already suffered from one heart attack, received counselling to reduce their Type A behaviour, they were less likely to suffer another attack as compared to similar persons who did not receive any counselling.

In spite of such positive results, the theory of a very defined personality type being a factor in heart disease lost ground throughout the 1980s giving way to the view that an inability to cope with stress was the major psychological contributor to heart disease. Individual differences in coping mechanisms, e.g., relaxation techniques, changes in diet, etc., came to play a larger part in attempts to reduce the incidence or recurrence of heart attacks.

Another interesting point is of course that some people cope very well under pressure and need such emotional highs to reach their work potential. (On a more facetious note, it is always possible that Type A individuals were really Type B people who had repressed their apathy and inertia so much as to create the opposite!) Through regular use of relaxation much can be achieved to change the tense approach to living adopted by highly stressed individuals prone to heart disease.

PERSONALITY PATTERNS AND CANCER

The following is a case history of someone whose cancer diagnosis led him to dealing with personality problems:

> Tom is a 70 year old retired builder who recently developed throat cancer. Only his wife and children were aware of the diagnosis. Tom is extremely intelligent and a very well read man whose one regret in life was that he never received a third level education. At 16, like his father and grandfather before him he began an apprenticeship as a carpenter. He was always very angry about this because he was given no choice in the matter. Some 10 years later he started his own business, but was never satisfied with his achievements because he was a perfectionist and overcritical. He built a beautiful home and his wife Kate was always supportive of his work. All his children received a good education and he was very proud of them. He was always trying to assess his purpose in life and his col-

leagues say that he is always putting himself down. Kate tried to keep the truth from him, but he eventually confronted her and she had to admit the diagnosis. Tom started reading everything he could find on cancer and became completely obsessed with finding a way to deal with his condition. He has started counselling and he is learning to deal with much 'un-finished business' from his childhood.

Environmental, dietary and physiological factors are other important factors, the presence of which can override the effects of personality on cancer. This does not however, take from the relevance of psychological factors and the importance of understanding the mental and emotional health, past and present, of each patient in their treatment.

Perhaps partly because cancer has become such a pervasive disease in our society, doctors are slow to consider the relevance of psychological factors in its onset. The medical professions' lack of control over such factors may be another reason why past psychological health is not often dealt with adequately in the treatment approach to cancer patients.

It is doubtful if a clear-cut cancer personality exists. However, there is some evidence that cancer patients are likely to have suffered severe emotional disturbance in their childhood (anytime up to the age of 15). This may be due to the breakdown/loss of parental relationships, divorce, death, illness, etc. As a child, such individuals may have suffered a great sense of loss, loneliness, anxiety and rejection.

In order to overcome the feeling of failure to form warm and satisfying relationships in childhood, these people make special efforts to overcompensate by trying constantly to please others and win their affection. If they do not succeed, they feel further loneliness, anger, helplessness and self-hatred. This in turn leads to anxiety and depression. In adult life, sometimes within six months to a year of the loss of a significant person or thing in their life, cancer appears. Their despair deepens when cancer is discovered and they are back into the helpless-hopeless mode of living again.

Treya Killam Wilbur in *Grace & Grit* described some of the traits linked to her cancer as follows:

- repressing emotions especially anger and sadness.
- significant life changes which cause stress and depression.
- being too self critical/perfectionist.
- a fatty diet with excess caffeine.
- struggling to define purpose in life.
- loneliness and hopelessness as a child, also an inability to express one's feelings as a child.
- overly independent and needing to be in control.
- inability to pursue a spiritual path in life.

The hypothesis that certain individuals may be psychologically predisposed to developing cancer is not new. The ancient physician Galen in 537 BC observed that 'melancholy' women were more likely to suffer from cancer than 'sanguine' women. Eighteenth and nineteenth century physicians noted a common thread running through all cancer victims, for example, despair, hopelessness following diverse occurrences such as death of a friend or relative, separation, economic, political or professional frustrations.

Stephanie Simonton, an American psychologist has become one of the most assertive authorities linking personality traits and cancer. In her book *The Healing Family*, she gives details of psychological studies which have identified a life history pattern which has led to hopelessness and low self-esteem in the typical cancer patient. One particular study she quotes, found that 76% of cancer patients felt isolated, neglected and despairing during their youth and early adulthood. Furthermore they bottled up their despair and did not communicate hurt, anger or hostility towards others.

Such evidence, according to Simonton, suggested that those who developed cancer had a life history of depression which led to chronic depression, lasting sometimes for twenty years or more, in which their feelings were suppressed. They were notably individuals who put other people first, because of their low self-esteem and who ignored their own needs. From such findings the Simonton approach encourages patients to be expressive with their anger and even to be 'selfish' as a way of increasing their self-esteem and bringing them out of themselves.

Dr Lawrence Le Shan found that in spite of their poor psychological health, cancer patients were often seen as wonderful people who were always smiling and pleasant. According to Le Shan, 'the benign qualities, the goodness of these people was in fact a sign of their failure to believe in themselves sufficiently and their lack of hope'.

Other studies by Thomas and Duszynski in the 1970s have found that cancer patients who seldom expressed strong emotion, were generally very 'low gear' and experienced a lack of closeness growing up.

The reason it is so important for someone with cancer to develop a more fulfilling, less stressful, emotional life, is that chronic depression and stress depress the immune response and speed up the progression of the cancer. According to Simonton there are no drugs or therapies as effective against cancer as the specific antigens an individual's body can create, through, for example, relaxation, complementary therapies such as aromatherapy, shiatsu, etc. The naturally produced antigens do much to release destructive toxins present in the body.

As we expressed at the beginning of this chapter, it is almost impossible to link a specified set of personality traits or a life history pattern to every cancer patient. The psychological dimension is only one factor in the complex aetiology of cancer.

PERSONALITY PATTERNS AND MIGRAINE

The following is a case history of someone who learned to deal with stress in her life as a solution to her frequent headaches:

> Jean is thirty years old. She has had classical migraine headaches since she was 15. In the beginning the headaches were usually associated with her monthly periods but as she went on in college she especially noticed that the headaches got worse each time she was due to sit her exams. Her GP suggested an elimination diet (which cut out food which triggered the headaches) i.e., cutting out pork, chocolate, dairy products such as cheese, spicy foods and red wine, which helped some what. But the real contributing factor is stress. Jean pushed herself very hard to relax until a friend suggested trying shiatsu therapy. Shiatsu therapy works on the energy meridians of the body thus stimulating relaxation and releasing the body of any damaging toxins. She says that since practising shiatsu, the frequency of her headaches have significantly reduced from about 2 hours a week to 2 headaches every 6 months. She also notices that she sleeps a lot better as well.

Some research suggests that patients whose doctors cannot find a physical cause for the migraine, have an initial psychological response of holding back from emotional involvement. They cease to let their emotional expression flow out towards other people and instead contain their anger and resentment. One of the effects of this habitual response, is the typical cold extremities sufferers experience at the onset of an attack. Sleep-onset insomnia usually follows if such emotional withdrawal continues.

Migraine headache can be a result of the disturbance of the tone of blood vessels in the head. Much research has shown that sufferers of migraine are more likely to possess Type A rather than Type B personality traits. They often feel unworthy, and they have great difficulty saying 'No' thus automatically take on more than they can cope with. Feelings of inadequacy lead to an incessant need for love and approval from other people.

Sufferers are accused of being rigid, somewhat self-righteous and at times fanatical. They push themselves hard and become impatient if others lag behind. They need to learn to address priority tasks and delegate tasks with more ease and less discomfort.

The greatest paradox of all is that most attacks occur during periods of leisure. It is as if the sufferer bottles up all his/her frustration and during so called 'relaxation time' all these emotions surface.

Having taken time out, (i.e., a period of undisturbed sleep) the symptoms of nausea, sensitivity to light and visual aberrations disappear. Stress management techniques such as a form of relaxation to be used every day, or a healthier diet have proved to be the most beneficial intervention for migraine sufferers over the last decade or so.

The followng case history shows how dealing with one's fears can help people cope with chronic conditions, such as arthritis.

> Anne is a 56 year old national schoolteacher. Anne's husband Mark describes her as a very tense, highly-strung, person who is a perfectionist. For the last 5 years Anne has suffered from rheumatoid arthritis. Despite several attempts at traditional interventions such as medication and physiotherapy, there has been little improvement. The rate of progression of her arthritis has been extremely fast since Anne was first diagnosed. Mark says she clearly went into depression and found the condition very difficult to accept. They have no children and Anne loves her job. Her greatest fear was of ending up an invalid like her grandmother. Mark brought Anne for counselling to help discuss her fears openly and at least at a psychological level there was a tremendous improvement.

Rheumatoid arthritis is known as an auto-immune disease in which the body 'turns in on itself'. It has puzzled researchers for several years whether or not a particular form of self-destructive personality translates into a self-destructive auto-immune disease.

In a study on 5,000 patients with rheumatoid arthritis as compared to a control group, rheumatoid patients were found to have a greater tendency to be self-sacrificing, masochistic, self-conscious, shy, inhibited and perfectionist than those in the control group. Female sufferers tended to be more nervous, tense and depressed and typically had mothers who they thought rejected them and fathers who were strict disciplinarians.

It is important to remember that such findings are only suggestive. The purpose of exploring these characteristics is not to alarm people who may exhibit some of the characteristics but to make them aware of their vulnerable behaviour patterns and under what conditions various illnesses are likely to show themselves.

SEX DIFFERENCES AND ILLNESS PATTERNS

In general, psychological studies have found that women turn their problems inwards, while men express their problems more publicly. For example, twice as many women as men suffer from depression, while more men turn to alcohol as a means of coping with their problems. Such differences can partly be explained through the social roles women and men have historically held. Having been more dominant in the workplace, the male problem surfacing is often alcoholism. While women have traditionally been linked more to the home, their problems tend to turn inwards, e.g., depression.

Research has also shown that in terms of physical illness, women suffer in larger numbers from such conditions as multiple sclerosis while men are more likely to develop heart conditions. The reasons for such differences are only explored in the heart disease literature. One explanation that has been offered to account for the sex difference in coronary rates relates to genetic differences. It is assumed that female sex hormones reduce cholesterol levels in the blood and thereby reduce the risk of heart disease. An-other variable that contributes to heart disease is smoking habits. Research has shown that more males smoke than females, although in some countries this is now changing.

Men are more likely to show strong Type A personality traits than their female counterparts. Some studies have shown that Type A females, although suffering less heart disease than Type A males, experience more heart disease than Type B males and Type B females. Women tend to live longer than men and their life expectancy continues to lengthen while men seem to be having shorter life spans. Perhaps one of the reasons for this may be the fact that more women go for treatment earlier than men.

- Enhance your coping skills by talking about your difficulties rather than taking everything on board yourself.
- Learn to express your anger by saying how you feel about something or somebody who may have hurt you.
- Overcome your feelings of rejection and enhance your self-esteem and your own abilities. List your positive personality traits on a daily basis.
- Start enjoying your own company, e.g. by listening to music, meditating, etc. This helps you to reduce your dependency on other people.
- Set yourself realistic time goals and avoid impatience, otherwise you will become aggressive and restless.
- Learn to say 'no' more often and you will discover that your overall productivity will improve.
- Remember we cannot all be good at everything, accept your limitations graciously. Do not allow your competitive nature to be destructive to you.
- Develop good time management skills by setting out a daily agenda for your recovery. Avoid a hyperactive approach to your lifestyle.
- Overcome your 'shyness' by participating in an

assertiveness training course.

- Remember you cannot control everything in your life. Be realistic and avoid perfectionism, by accepting your limits.

5

HOW SUCCESSFUL IS DRUG TREATMENT?

Everything is a dangerous drug to me except reality, which is unendurable.
CYRIL CONNOLLY

How have drugs become so commonplace in the treatment of illness? What is a placebo drug and how powerful are its psychological effects in relieving pain symptoms? How important are psychological factors in the treatment of illness?

From a very early age when we are sick or feeling unwell, we expect the doctor or one of our parents to give us some medicine to take our pain away. We learn as young children to adopt a passive rather than an active role in the treatment of our illnesses. In later life, many patients become so keen to be treated with drugs that they are critical of general practitioners who refuse to prescribe medication and suggest alternative coping techniques instead. Some such patients get caught up in a special language of drugs and treatment which separates them from their bodies. The result can be that they lose their identity in the process of becoming ill and feel that their bodies do not belong to them but to the doctors.

Many older patients get a strange satisfaction from showing their various tablets for insomnia, arthritis, blood pressure, fluid retention, etc., to their family and friends. The more medication they have, the greater they believe their chances are of being 'cured'. They sit back and wait for the tablets to take their course. If this is not immediate, they will sometimes dangerously experiment with a complete cocktail of drugs before they feel they have found the right one. Often, they don't really know which medication is treating which symptoms but they are happy to be taking their tablets. Always listen to what your doctor advises and do not experiment.

People have always used chemicals to alter their states of consciousness and to change their behaviour. In primitive societies, plants that influenced perception and consciousness were eaten or inhaled. Witch doctors had a whole plethora of 'magic cures' and potions. Even the fathers of modern medicine, Hippocrates and Galen used medicines with several hundred ingredients, many of whose curative effects were not clearly known.

Since the 1950s we have moved from a predominantly drug-free society to a drug-dependent society. In many ways, the increased use of drugs began when such wonder drugs as penicillin first became available. In the 1930s and 1940s, antibiotics and sulpha drugs were introduced and people came to realise that these drugs could be used to help diseased bodies return to their normal healthy state.

In the 1950s, the major and minor tranquillisers became widely used in the treatment of emotional problems and mental illness. People learned that drugs could help a diseased mind (e.g., a psychiatric condition such as depression) return to normal, just as other drugs helped diseased bodies. In the 1960s oral contraceptives first appeared in the market-place and many healthy women began taking these hormonal drugs to prevent them from becoming pregnant.

Much too was learned about investigative procedures before safely allowing drugs on the market. Many mistakes were made and several drugs such as slimming tablets (e.g., MER 29) and Thalidomide (originally taken to help with morning sickness during pregnancy and later found to cause physical abnormalities in babies) were withdrawn. More recently controversy exists around the anti-depressant Ativan and some patients have experienced adverse effects from the new anti-depressant, Prozac.

Drug use increased through the 1970s and early 1980s as an increasing number of illegal drugs such as marijuana, the hallucinogens, stimulants and sedatives became available. While a downward trend of drug abuse appeared in the mid 1980s, this is believed to have risen again in the 1990s.

Drug addiction has become a very real problem in our society whether it be the hidden abuse of sedatives, anti-depressants and over the counter medicines or the more public problem of heroin or cocaine addiction.

A PLACEBO DRUG

Most of what we know about how drugs act on our system has been learned through studies using placebos. A placebo is a physiologically inert medication that still may cause an effect through the psychological factor of suggestibility. If the patient expects to feel better or is told by an authority figure (e.g., a doctor, nurse or parent) that their condition is likely to improve, then it often does so regardless of the inert quality of their medication.

Medicines used by Hippocrates and Galen were placebos. In their studies, both physicians noted that people with greater levels of confidence in their methods had more successful prognoses. Nowadays, between 50% to 80% of all symptoms of illness are considered to have some emotional as well as physical content. Different researchers have found that up to 45% of patients claim pain relief having taken placebo medication.

Most forms of medical treatment rely on the placebo effect to some extent. Antibiotics, vitamins and surgery have a placebo component which in some cases may account for any improvement – it is not necessarily the chemical content of the drug that causes change but it may be the fact that a change is expected as a result of taking medication or other forms of intervention. Some orthopaedic consultants believe in the placebo effect of physiotherapy. A patient's perception that intervention will in some way improve their condition can actually lead to a reported improvement in general well-being and quality of life.

Many doctors have wonderful anecdotes of complaining patients who were quietened by the injections of sterile water or glasses of sugary water. The following is one such example encountered:

'I can remember one very busy Friday afternoon when I was working in an out-patient's clinic. A patient came into a clinic. He was complaining that he was bored waiting to see the consultant. He began to shout and scream with pain. One of the staff went into the hospital kitchen and mixed a glass of sugar and water. She came out and told him to drink it and his pain would disappear. He suddenly became more subdued – much to everyone's relief in the clinic – and thanked the staff member sincerely for her help.'

The late Dr Henry K. Beecher, anaesthesiologist at Harvard University, discovered that 35% of patients consistently experienced satisfactory relief when placebos were used instead of regular medication for a wide range of medical problems including severe post-operative pain, sea-sickness, headaches, coughs and anxiety. Other

biological processes and disorders improved by placebos, as reported by medical researchers, include rheumatoid and degenerative arthritis, blood-cell count, respiratory problems, hay fever and hypertension.

The fact that a placebo will have no physiological
effect if the patient knows it is a placebo, only confirms
something about the capacity of the human body to
transform hope into tangible and essential biochemical
change. Current speculation suggests that the effects of
placebos are mediated through the body's natural pain
killing enzymes known as endorphins. Endorphins
which are often dubbed the brain's opiates, affect how
the individual subjectively experiences pain and mood.
It is thought that they are produced when one expects to
become well and better able to cope.

Since medicine has begun to take on a more multi-
disciplinary approach (with psychologists, physiotherapists, dieticians, acupuncturists, etc.) it is now becoming
more and more difficult to attribute all change reported
by a patient to drug intervention alone. Doctors and
health care professionals recognise the need to see the
patient as more than a set of 'walking symptoms'. The
patient has emotions and beliefs all of which will influence the success of treatment.

If a patient's confidence is built up by the use of a
placebo for example, he/she will feel safer and less
stressed about further treatment. This has been shown in
several patients receiving chemotherapy and elective
surgery. When an anaesthetist comes in to talk to a
patient before an operation (to explain the anaesthetic
procedure), this reduces the patient's anxiety levels significantly.

Here is a case history of a patient who benefited from
psychological counselling to help her make up her mind

to decide on having chemotherapy and on the administration of drugs, including a placebo drug, to reduce post-chemotherapy vomiting.(The patient was unaware while taking the drugs which was the placebo as she had previously given consent to partake in a research project.)

Audrey is a 35 year old woman who had breast cancer. She was advised by her consultant to start chemotherapy as soon as possible. Audrey struggled with the decision to accept or reject chemotherapy. She said, 'In the beginning I was almost certain that I would refuse it because I think poisoning one's body is an extremely crude way of dealing with cancer, and in many cases, its effectiveness can be called into question'. She requested some time to make her decision and she and her husband David decided to spend a week at a complementary clinic for cancer patients. During the week she learned relaxation techniques, had intensive counselling sessions, and participated in music therapy, art therapy, journalling and spiritual healing sessions while also seeing an orthodox doctor, a dietician and a Chinese medicine expert. There were also several group sessions where participants learned to express their feelings to a group, and how to change aspects of their lives that had been detrimental to them.

The therapy focused on helping the patients to come to terms with their conditions, to make them responsible for their own health in the future, and to learn to express the negative emotions that they had so carefully buried since childhood. Audrey said 'as the week progressed, and the therapy began to work, one by one we got in touch with our feelings. It was quite moving. One patient steadfastly insisted that her life was perfect in every way, that there was nothing she would want to change, but by the end of the week, the protective shell she had built around herself was beginning to crack. I had my first counselling session on Monday night and immediately the floodgates opened.

'As the week passed, we began our relaxation classes (which I badly needed), and during one session, we were mentally led up a winding mountain road, until we arrived at the cottage of a wise old woman. We had to ask her one question which was uppermost in our minds at that moment, and mine of course was: "Should I have chemo?" Instead of answering verbally, she gave each of us a symbol (which we all chose ourselves), and mine was a red rose, because it's my favourite flower.

'Later we had to draw the symbol with crayons, and it wasn't until I came to draw the thorns that I realised the significance of it. The wise old woman was of course my inner self, and the rose was symbolic of a bright future, free of cancer. The thorns, however brought home to me the fact that in order to achieve this state, I must also accept the sting. I am the type of person, who if I refused chemotherapy and the cancer returned, would be so wrapped up in guilt and self-blame, that there would be no energy left to fight the disease. If, however, I accepted the chemotherapy and at the same time changed some of the elements and attitudes in my life that allowed the cancer to flourish in the first place, I would have more peace of mind and could remain vigilant without becoming obsessive. Should it return, I could then devote all my strength and energy towards destroying it once again.

'Anyway that is how I reached my decision to go ahead with the chemo, and I'm still reeling from the shock because before the counselling I truly felt I would reject it.'

As soon as Audrey returned she began chemotherapy. Her greatest fear was of constant post-chemotherapy vomiting. Placebos and anti-nausea drugs were successfully administered by her oncologist and vomiting was greatly minimised. The multi-disciplinary approach to her treatment helped her to be more at ease and to respond better.

PSYCHOLOGICAL PREPARATION FOR MEDICAL AND SURGICAL TREATMENT

There is now abundant evidence in the medical/psychological literature that taking particular care over psychological preparation for medical and surgical procedures improves recovery on a wide range of criteria. Such preparation reduces the patient's distress and the length of hospitalisation. One of the clearest demonstrations of the value of preparation for surgery was reported by the English anaesthetist Egbert. He had two groups of patients one who received routine hospital information and the other who received practical information including how to cope post-operatively, how to deal with complications, etc. Those who received the extra practical advice experienced less anger, resentment and discomfort after their operation. They were rated by staff as making a quicker recovery. They required less post-operative medication and were discharged on average three days sooner. Dr Moore-Groarke repeated this study in 1989 on elderly cataract patients and found similar results.

Psychological variables are also important in rehabilitation. How much pain patients will experience and how long they will be absent from work are both predictable from their level of anxiety and depression about their illness. There is encouraging evidence showing that providing patients with help in adjusting to their illness improves their prospects for rehabilitation. Health psychology plays an important role in the rehabilitation of cardiac patients by teaching them more appropriate life skills and life changes.

DOCTOR – PATIENT RELATIONSHIP

Treatment compliance is also an important area for health psychology to consider. A high proportion of medical patients are prescribed medication, but the effects obviously depend on whether the patients actually take the medication prescribed. Advice given to patients about prevention and recovery must be put into practice to be effective.

If a patient is happy with a doctor, he or she is more likely to follow medical advice and comply with treatment. Studies have shown that in-patients are most likely to follow their treatments while out-patients show poorest compliance. The implication is that if supervision is increased, compliance is also increased. The following case history highlights this point. The patient's family can also help and patients can be visited by the public health nurse.

Health psychologists now play an important role in encouraging patients to comply with treatment regimes. Psychological procedures designed to increase patients co-operation are almost universally applicable and have paid significant dividends in health care.

Anne-Marie is a young overweight patient with a history of coronary heart disease. She was told that unless she lost weight she would have another heart attack. She agreed with her GP to go into hospital for 3 weeks to lose weight, under the supervision of a physician. Her in-patient programme was successful and she lost 14 pounds in weight.

For the next 3 months she attended the hospital one day a week to follow their dietary programme and attended their out-patient clinic for six months. Once discharged from hospital, Anne-Marie found it extremely difficult to control her diet. She was in control the days she returned to the hospital but she made very little progress as an out-patient. It was only when she revealed to the doctor that there was a problem of domestic violence at home did she start to make any progress. She had to be re-admitted for a second in-patient stay. Her physician referred her to the hospital's psychiatrist to work on the relevant issues behind her overeating.

ADVICE TO PEOPLE ON SEEING THEIR DOCTORS
The following are a list of points that patients should note, in order to improve the communication channels between doctor and patient.

1. Ask your doctor not to use technical language. Ask him/her to explain your condition, treatment, etc., in an easy to understand manner. The way a professional expresses him/herself when talking to you is very important. Technical terms mean nothing to you if you are in pain and fearful of an impending procedure or awaiting test results. Geriatric patients express the most difficulty when technical language is used, and often are afraid to ask for procedures to be explained.

2. Do not be afraid to ask questions – Although it may sometimes seem like a waste of time, it is very important for your well-being that the health care professional provides an atmosphere in which you can feel free to ask questions. Write down your questions beforehand and do not make any apologies, it is your right to ask for clarification.

Research has shown that when patients understand their illness better, they feel less anxiety and are less likely to have post-operative complications. Fear or feelings of discomfort with asking questions indicates a poor doctor-patient relationship. Assertive patients are far more likely to ask questions. Most people fear they will ask the wrong questions or that they will be laughed at. Medical schools are now teaching young doctors better communication skills with patients. In the United States and recently in Ireland the introduction of patient charters have put greater pressure on doctors to take time out and discuss with patients their fears and anxieties.

Sample questions:
It is necessary for me to take medication? Can I be referred for a second opinion? Are there any complications associated with the prescribed medication? How soon should I start to feel an improvement? What do you feel is my long term prognosis? Is hospital my only choice?

3. Take a sense of responsibility in your recovery – Many people seek help because they feel they have lost control over the difficulties in their lives and also because they believe it is the responsibility of the 'professional' to alleviate their problems. This is especially true of chronic pain patients. It is therefore important that the patient takes some of this responsibility for his/her recovery

4. Be aware of the psychological component in illness – All illnesses are the result of environmental, social, psychological and physiological factors. It is important for all health care professionals to

understand the significance of each factor in individual cases. By learning to recognise that thoughts, feelings and behaviours have an influence on their physical conditions, patients are likely to assume more responsibility for their treatment and can in some cases require less drug intervention. Some doctors may be reluctant to make a referral for psychological or complementary treatment. Stress to him/her that this is a possible option you are aware of/interested in, and it is your choice to explore all avenues in your road to leading a full life.

Accessing lifestyle issues, stress and personal well-being are all important for full recovery. Relaxation techniques as discussed in the following chapter are also important when recovering from or coping with a serious illness.

6

PSYCHOLOGICAL INTERVENTION IN COPING WITH ILLNESS

Doctors don't know everything really. They understand matter, not spirit.
And you and I live in the spirit.
WILLIAM SAROYAN, *THE HUMAN COMEDY*

What are the healing messages we can give ourselves? What are the most common psychological intervention techniques? Are there any plans that will help us to stay well? What is the role of complementary medicine?

The medical profession is learning that disease cannot be fully understood unless the person who has the disease is understood. Up to recently the 'diseased' person was seen purely as a set of walking symptoms. Thankfully, there is an increased awareness within the medical profession that good doctor-patient communication can enhance a patient's overall recovery. The patient is now seen as a complex person with a physical, mental, emotional, social and spiritual aspects to his/her personality.

The American doctor, Bernie Siegal has devoted his writings and research to the belief that we, the patients, play a major role in our own recovery, and at the same time acknowledges the necessity of medical intervention. In his work he makes an important distinction between, being healed and being cured. He says that to be healed represents a condition of one's life, while to be cured relates strictly to one's physical condition, excluding one's mental and emotional well-being. Being 'cured' is viewing people only as walking symptoms. For example parents often ask, 'when will my daughter be cured of anorexia?' In a traditional medical approach the patient is cured once they reach a target weight for age, height, sex and build and in the case of a female patient is menstruating regularly. Any professional knows that to measure the person's progress only in this respect ignores the many factors of an emotional nature behind the condition.

Siegal also makes the point that there is no disease whose treatment cannot be enhanced by a doctor who knows how to inspire and guide patients to encourage the body's internal healers. He stresses active rather than passive participation by the patient. Doctors nowadays are more ready to recognise that they are merely facilitators or catalysts of healing, not the healers.

Patients should focus on their need to make necessary changes to improve their overall quality of life, rather than on the fact that the doctor emphasised that they smoked, lived a sedentary lifestyle, had high cholesterol, etc. Adapting to necessary life changes can be difficult initially. A smoker will experience a certain withdrawal if he/she decides to stop smoking, and they may become irritable or moody if they are requested to change their diet. As well they may feel that such changes means losing a certain amount of their independence. Often patients describe feelings of 'surrender' to their illness. The word 'surrender' is commonly used in illnesses, of an addictive nature, e.g., alcoholism, bulimia nervosa. In both these examples patients describe how they surrender to drink, bingeing and purging respectively. A good support mechanism is vital to help guide the patient out of the sickness role. This support is best received from family and friends, but it is also helps to talk to patients who are well into recovery. It is also advisable for the family to learn all they can about their loved one's disease or illness. Educating oneself increases awareness and helps one know what to expect. The carers should not be afraid to ask for help for themselves.

AS IN ALL HUMAN experience, individuals and families react differently to illness depending on whether the condition in question has touched their lives previously. The same factors that influence one's reaction to pain (see chapter 3) come into play when someone is faced with either a chronic or acute illness.

The knowledge or lack of knowledge of the prognosis is one of the strongest influencing factors on an individual's ability to cope well with an illness or not. Sometimes the recurrence of a hereditary condition such as a heart attack can send panic waves through an entire family whereas in other cases when a cancer is identified for the first time, the family's coping strategies can be pulled into place to help 'rally round' the sick member.

The psychological techniques dealt with in the following pages can be of help to the healthy members of the family as well as the person suffering from a particular illness. Some of the ideas in the 10 point plan for the control of pain in Chapter 3 can also be useful for carers of the sick or family members who are particularly stressed due to the illness of a spouse, son or daughter.

PSYCHOLOGICAL TECHNIQUES

Stress inoculation training
This bizarre sounding technique is used by psychologists in health care settings throughout the western world. It

was first proposed by the psychologist Meichenbaum in the mid 1970s. It is based on the principle that people can be taught to change their 'internal dialogue' as a psychological aid to reduce stress levels and the physical symptoms of ill health.

The theory is that each individual's inner speech can be positive or negative. If patients' perception of their condition improves, they become much more positive and confident about their own healing ability. Such a belief is crucial for patients to play an active role in recovery from illness or disease.

Anyone who engages in stress inoculation training follows a specific programme which begins with an explanation of how positive and negative thinking can influence their physical health as well as their mental and emotional well-being. The goal of stress inoculation training is to train the patient to talk to him/herself differently about the problem. Patients are encouraged to analyse their problems instead of reacting in a panicky way or resigning themselves to suffering.

When patients adopt a fear reaction towards their illness, two specific processes begin. First there is an increase in physiological arousal, for example increased heart rate, sweaty palms, rapid breathing and body tension. Second, anxiety engendering thoughts increase – images and self-statements such as I'm nervous or I'm sweating replace positive statements such as I'm in control or I am relaxed.

These reactions are explained to the patient who is then taught to use the physiological and psychological cues associated with the stress response to trigger a variety of coping responses. Although this theory sounds like the power of positive thinking advocated in many popular books, its advice is much more specific, dealing with how individuals can change their behaviour in a precise and directed manner.

In stress inoculation training patients are instructed in the use of specific phrases or affirmations, for example, 'I am relaxed', 'I can feel the tension disappear', 'I too can help heal my body', and behavioural skills, 'I am choosing to give up smoking', 'I acknowledge the need to change my diet', 'I look forward to my daily walk', etc., and are advised to practise these skills regularly.

Each set of phrases and each behaviour skill is specific to the patients' condition and circumstances. This technique has been found to be useful in the treatment of diseases such as colitis, irritable bowel syndrome, recurrent abdominal pain and nervous diarrhoea.

Stress inoculation training is now taught as a part of most stress management courses, to help with the prevention of disease or to control addictive behaviour. Many ante-natal classes teach this technique combined with relaxation to help in the early stages of labour. Lou Tice in Seattle uses this technique for people in business.

The following is a case history of someone who learned to use positive inner speech:

> Aileen was in her 40s when she first came for treatment. For a number of years she suffered from nervous diarrhoea. It started when her husband's business went bankrupt, and she was left to face the banks, creditors, liquidators, etc. Her husband Dan opted out by signing himself into a psychiatric institution.
>
> Her first memory of having an attack was the day she had to go into the bank manager and plead with him not to take the family home but instead to allow them to remortgage it. Aileen grew up in an environment where money was plentiful and she never had to face anything like this before. She was recommended to see a psychologist by her GP who consequently put her on a stress inoc-

ulation training programme. The primary aim of the programme was to help Aileen to relax. She was taught some simple breathing techniques and encouraged to use positive rather than negative inner speech. She was given 3 affirmations (positive statements) to practise daily whether she felt under stress or not. Soon she started to feel more relaxed and the diarrhoea disappeared altogether within 2 months. The affirmations were as follows:

(a) I release myself of all my anxieties and fly as free as a bird,

(b) I am choosing to take control of my life and discharge myself of playing the role of passive wife, mother, lover and friend,

(c) I can heal my body, and my problem will disappear.

Biofeedback

In the 1970s we were bombarded with claims that many illnesses from the common cold to cancer were treatable through a new self-control technique called biofeedback. In the United States, many patients rushed out to buy the electronically controlled monitoring devices which recorded and displayed physiological processes within the body.

The most successful clinical applications of biofeedback were found in sufferers of high blood pressure and headaches. 5% to 10% of the general population suffer from high blood pressure and the use of biofeedback over time was found to improve their conditions substantially. The severity and frequency of tension and migraine headaches was also significantly reduced through biofeedback. Many neurology clinics still teach biofeedback. Epilepsy is another condition which benefited from biofeedback.

The effectiveness of biofeedback may simply be due to the fact that it enables patients to focus on their physiological condition. Their motivation to have better readings on the monitor plays a contributing role. Such a process says a lot about the links between the mind and the body.

The following is a case history of how one individual used biofeedback to reduce her high blood pressure:

Gill was in her early 30s when she was expecting her first child. Thirty-six weeks into the pregnancy she started to develop high blood pressure. The problem is that high blood pressure can lead to toxaemia which can, if allowed to progress, lead to an emergency caesarean section instead of a vaginal delivery. Gill's gynaecologist was very progressive and suggested she try biofeedback 3 times a day over 10 days and if there was an improvement he would allow the pregnancy to full term. Gill and her husband were taught how to use the monitor and she was also taught how to practise deep breathing. Each time Gill's blood pressure increased, the monitor would echo this by making a loud noise. Once Gill disciplined herself to using the monitor the next ante-natal check up recorded that her blood pressure had returned to normal. She later delivered at 39 weeks vaginally.

Meditation

Although the most popular form of meditation in this country is Transcendental Meditation or TM, some individuals also practise meditation through yoga and martial arts. The technique is very simple and involves sitting comfortably with your eyes closed twice a day for approximately twenty minutes. During that time, you think or repeat a Sanskrit sound or mantra. Mantras are selected for each individual by an instructor. Thoughts are allowed to drift into mind and then are released or 'thrown away'. Eventually calm and peacefulness replaces ones customary busy 'mind chatter'.

Meditation has been found to have a calming effect on those who practise it regularly. Many believe that one of the main reasons for its success is due to the fact that the individual starts to assume more responsibility for his/her health. Meditation has had useful clinical applications in the treatment of hypertension, insomnia, headaches and asthma.

The following is a case history of someone who successfully used meditation to deal with her neck pain:

> Serena presented with a recurring pain down the back of her neck and right shoulder. Numerous medical investigations revealed nothing of a physical nature to explain her symptoms. Her doctor who was extremely vigilant noticed that Serena was a rather tense person and suggested she see a therapist. The therapist taught her some basic yoga technique which helped the body to relax. This was followed by some Shiatsu massage (acupressure on energy meridians of the body). In the space of 6 weeks, Serena was symptom free. Obviously what was happening was that Serena's stress was manifesting itself in physical pain in her neck and shoulder.

Visualisation

Visualisations are a particular kind of meditation which makes use of imagery. Using visualisations, individuals put their imagination to work to create images of what they are trying to achieve. Such visualisations have been found to be effective preparations for goals ranging from improved sports performance to natural childbirth. They can be hypnotically induced or self induced but, whichever way, it is important that individuals are allowed to supply their own personal imagery. Once again the patients active involvement is important.

The following exercise is a summary of Carl Simonton's method, where he encourages us to utilise our natural physical defences through visualisation.

1. Relax in a comfortable chair with your feet on the floor and your extremities supported so that they are not strained. Ensure quiet, a comfortable room temperature and soft lighting.
2. Use a simple relaxation exercise by breathing in and out very slowly for a minute or so, described in chapter 2.
3. Relax in your special place for a few minutes.
4. Create a mental picture of your illness or injury. Imagine it in a form that makes sense to you. If you have a broken arm, you could imagine the jagged ends of the bone roughly meeting but not attached. If you have a stomach ulcer, you might see an inflamed, raw sore on the stomach wall.
5. Picture a treatment – magical or scientific – that will eliminate the injury or illness, or strengthen your body's ability to heal itself. If you are under treatment you can visualise it working effectively. Imagine seeing your broken bone resting peacefully, enclosed in a protective case. Imagine milk or antacids coating the ulcer with soothing, healing white liquid that neutralises the acid and reduces the inflammation.
6. Picture your natural physical defences and physical processes eliminating the illness or injury. See new, red blood flowing in, multiplying and forming a thick, gluey substance that binds the pieces of bone together. See healthy cells multiplying and covering the ulcer, and white blood cells removing the debris and cleansing the area.
7. See yourself as healthy and free from illness, injury

and pain. See your bone completely healed, stronger than ever. See yourself participating in your favourite activities, feeling happy, healthy and pain free. See your stomach lining pink and healthy. See yourself feeling calm and vital, enjoying yourself.

8. See yourself successfully proceeding toward achieving the goals in your life. See yourself participating in your career, in sports, in your community. See yourself with a healthy, happy family. See yourself taking a trip you have long wanted to take.

9. Congratulate yourself for participating in your own recovery. See yourself doing this exercise three times a day in a relaxed and alert state.

(Reprinted with permission by New Harbringer Publications, Inc., Oakland, California.)

The following case history is an example of how one woman used visualisation successfully:

Denise suffered from respiratory problems. While in therapy she was asked to visualise herself as a river. The therapist guided her into examining what kind of a river she saw herself as – a long, narrow, winding, twisting, river with streams or tributaries? What was the bank of the river like? Were there fish in the river, algae, etc.

Denise imagined her river to be overgrown with algae in bloom. Everything that fell into her river was smothered or experienced feelings of suffocation. She describes a deep sense of falling deeper and deeper on entering the river. In psychotherapy, she addressed these emotions triggered by the visualisation technique. It turned out that Denise nearly drowned when she was 5 years old and had since developed a phobia for water. The therapist later introduced her to a pleasant image of a river which helped release her fears and some time later her respiratory problems disappeared because as soon as the feelings of suffocation at an emotional level were under control they also ceased at a physical level.

Relaxation

An English psychologist in the 1930s, Edmond Jacobsen was the first to introduce progressive relaxation in a medical context based on yoga techniques. The physiology of the relaxation response is what distinguishes it from what we usually mean when we talk about relaxing. The relaxation response is much more than sitting down watching a favourite television programme or reading an interesting book. The body both feels and is in better balance when the relaxation response is evoked. Physiologically, heart rate, general metabolism, oxygen consumption and respiration slow down, blood pressure and muscle tension are lowered and brain activity is characterised by alpha waves which are slower in frequency than what is usual in a waking state.

Regular or structured relaxation is an excellent form of preventative medicine and can be used before the onset of any illness or disease as part of an overall routine for an enhanced quality of life. Relaxation can also be used with visualisation as discussed earlier in this chapter.

The clinical applications of relaxation are numerous. Relaxation has been shown to be helpful to cardiac patients. In the United States, psychologist Joan Bortsenko showed that many diabetics are able to use relaxation to reduce the need and frequency of insulin use. Relaxation training has also helped asthma sufferers and patients with chronic and acute pain.

Relaxation training can also take place in a group

therapy setting where it is a useful strategy for encouraging attitude and behaviour change necessary for recovery. Dr Moore-Groarke's own research has shown that relaxation can reduce the frequency and severity of migraine headaches and that daily relaxation can reduce the frequency of self-induced purging episodes in bulimic patients.

The following case history shows how relaxation helped one man to give up smoking:

> John was a heavy smoker for 15 years. A recent trip to his GP revealed another bout of bronchitis and John was urged to stop smoking. John made several attempts to stop but failed. On hearing that John smoked to 'help him relax' the GP suggested he learn relaxation and practise it daily. At first John was dubious about this but was prepared at least to give it a try for 2 weeks. The first week was very difficult but during the second week John was now familiar with using the relaxation technique so each time he felt like a cigarette, he started to use the relaxation breathing. He is now off cigarettes 6 months and is positive for the future.

Systematic desensitisation/Aversion therapy

Developed by Dr Joseph Wolpe in the 1950s, systematic desensitisation is a stress management technique that can be used by those preparing for surgery. The individual is helped to imagine stressful scenes such as the operating room while in a profound state of relaxation. By progressively imagining more and more stressful scenes while relaxed, the individual learns to face these situations without incapacitating anxiety. The individual can thus rehearse such techniques. This technique is most widely used in the treatment of phobias where a person imagines different stages of confronting their phobic reaction (e.g., to spiders, dogs, cats) in a relaxed state.

The following is an example of how aversion therapy was used to help a patient deal with alcohol cravings:

> Aidan is an alcoholic. As part of his treatment programme he took part in a systematic desensitisation programme that his psychiatrist worked out with him. Each time he experienced a craving to drink he was asked firstly to imagine himself falling off the barstool on tasting a drink, secondly being on the floor and getting sick and thirdly of being unable to stop vomiting every time he tried to drink from the glass. This technique started to become effective after 6 weeks. He was taught to become desensitised to the pleasures he once associated with drinking. The pleasures were replaced with feelings of aversion. Of course this approach was not the only approach used with Aidan. Aidan also had intense psychotherapy and relaxation skills training but systematic desensitisation was extremely helpful in helping him to deal with cravings.

RECOVERY PLAN

This recovery plan will be of help to anyone recovering from an illness or accident – when they must spend some time in convelescence.

1. Do things in life that bring a sense of joy and fulfilment. Much time is spent doing things that have to be done ... Create fun in your life. Do things that you have always wanted to do and visit places that you have always wanted to visit. Many patients only travel abroad when they discover that they have only a short time left to live.

2. Pay close attention to your needs. A hierarchy of needs, developed by Abraham Maslow has become a tool for many psychologists in explaining the importance for basic needs like food, water and shelter to be satisfied before other emotional

and mental needs can be fulfilled. Patients make a list of their immediate needs and identify needs in the future, e.g., significance of their condition, recovery, etc.

3. Release negative emotions, e.g., anger, hostility. Once a choice is made negative emotions can be easily replaced by positive ones. A useful exercise is to make a list of people you have being angry with in your life. State why and how the anger affected you.

4. Hold positive images in your mind. Positive images include walking on a sea-shore, being in your favourite place, etc.

5. Love yourself and everyone else. Although this sounds like a very charismatic notion, love is a very important emotion to believe in on a conscious level. Believing in your own value and self-worth is the necessary starting point before you can reach out with such positive feelings to other people. By loving yourself, you stop judging yourself and other people. Practise positive affirmations such as, e.g., 'I am feeling better and better'.

6. Create fun in your life by being spontaneous. Dr Moore-Groarke had a patient once who took a parachute jump in the hope of releasing his mind from destructive thoughts.

7. Make a positive contribution to the community. Perhaps you could start by joining a support group, doing some charity work, talk to the media about how you have helped yourself. Remember there is always someone less fortunate than you.

8. Make a commitment to health and well-being and

develop a belief in total health. Many people have the misconception that disease is a form of punishment. Disease can be a gift which can help us transform our lives.

9. Accept yourself and everything in your life as an opportunity for growth and learning. This is hard at first but by talking to those who are in recovery they will tell you that when you no longer take life for granted, this is a wonderful step forward.

10. Keep a sense of humour, see the funny side of your illness, e.g., if you have to wear a temporary wig because of chemotherapy, change your hairstyle in the wig.

Complementary medicine

It has become increasingly clear, both to the medical establishment and the general public, that alternative/complementary forms of medicine make a positive contribution to health care today. The term 'alternative' is confusing. We have a preference for the word complementary, as it is used to cover many diverse approaches to healing.

Very simply, treatments fall into three categories:

(A) Structural therapies – for example, chiropractic and osteopathy, deal in the physical manipulation of body parts to rectify physical injury or maladjustment.

(B) Vital force therapies – these therapies adopt a more subtle approach and probe deeper into the whole symptom/lifestyle picture, e.g., yoga, aromatherapy, reflexology, acupuncture.

(C) Psychotherapies – for example, psychotherapy, counselling and hypnotherapy.

A good guide to complementary medicine is Margot McCarthy's 1995 guide *Natural therapies – The Complete A-Z Guide of Complementary Health*. She makes the point that health should be a personal responsibility. The reason for the growth of psychological medicine and complementary medicine is that people now realise that disease has to be seen within the context of one's entire life. Disease forces people to appraise their complete lifestyle.

In choosing the right therapy, once the therapist is sure that the patient has been checked by a doctor to make certain that the symptoms do not mask an underlying medical problem, it can be useful to set up or arrange for an advisory session. During the advisory session, there are says three main points that need to be addressed according to Margot McCarthy:

(1) Ascertaining the cause of the main problem, in other words is the problem primarily mental, physical or emotional.
(2) Looking at the patient as a 'whole' and not fragmenting the patient's complaint from other areas of his/her life.
(3) Selecting the optimum treatment available for that particular individual not just for the complaint.

Sometimes, one or more complementary technique will be recommended. Individuals should discuss any reservations they have with the therapist. Some techniques of complementary health care will be better known to you than others.

According to an English psychologist, Andrew Stanway, what has also helped modern medicine is society's improvements such as good sanitation, improved housing, smaller families and other social improvements. The increase in life expectancy cannot be accredited to medicine alone. However, he stresses that certain drug innovations, e.g., antibiotics have made a difference. The rise in stress-related disorders for example depression, anxiety and chronic fatigue, and the disease of 'being in a hurry' are very much a sign of the times and require a multi-disciplinary intervention programme. Psychology and complementary health care will continue to play a significant role in treatment programmes around the world. It is exciting to see also the number of clinical applications of such therapies increasing.

7

CREATING A BETTER WAY

No one is a failure who is enjoying life.

ANON.

Creating a better way, means facing up to the psychological, emotional and physical challenges that life can bring. For many people the traditional medical model of treatment of illness is sufficient. For several others, an approach which includes the skills of alternative practices or a combination of the two is most beneficial. An anonymous quotation in 1855 asks the question – 'Is life worth living? That depends on the liver'. The poet Longfellow in his writings on a psalm for life sums up our ability to create a better way as follows 'Life is real! Life is earnest! And the grave is not its goal'.

The importance of a positive mental attitude and emotional maturity in recovery has been established through numerous research projects and personal experiences. Many sick people also come out of their illness with a better self-knowledge and understanding of human nature which in turn helps them return to full health with a different attitude towards themselves and others. Coping strategies such as vigilance (i.e., facing up to one's illness) need to be learned and practised. In the early stages of illness when many people are in denial they choose to adopt an avoidance coping strategy. If this strategy is prolonged, it delays the inevitable challenge that faces all patients, and consequently leads to depression.

Social connectness or closeness to other people is also a good ally for those recovering from an illness. Having someone who you can be honest with and rely on relieves many burdens, allowing him/her to concentrate on getting better. Much research on eating disordered patients has shown that those with poor family support are slower to recover. Dr Moore-Groarke's research has shown that those whose families refuse to attend for family therapy are less likely to recover quickly because nothing has changed within the family dynamics. To recover you need to change your attitude if you cannot change your situation. A listening ear often is the key to recovery alone. Requests for medication are also greater among the patients who have nobody to talk to about their illness. The hospital psychologist/counsellor has a very valuable role to play here with such patients. Some hospitals in Ireland provide pastoral care (with a spiritual guidance) and many patients find great comfort in this.

The greatest difficulties are when the sufferers wear down the carers. The question that arises is 'who cares for the carers?' Several support groups (many of whom we have listed in our section useful addresses at the back of the book) recognise this factor.

Some helpful hints to carers are as follows:

(1) In order to help other people you need to be feeling well yourself, i.e., at a physical and emotional level. Always look after your own health.
(2) Set limits to the time you spend with the person you are caring for. Plan that you have additional support to facilitate some time off.
(3) Recruit others who are willing to help, otherwise the entire onus will fall on you.
(4) Never be afraid to say 'no'. Boundaries are extreme-

ly important – otherwise you will feel used and taken for granted.

(5) Get to know the doctor, or public health nurse, of the person you are caring for. Build up a rapport so that if you are having difficulties you can discuss them with the professionals. Sometimes patients will pay more attention to their nurse or doctor than the 'carer' they see every day.

Now we will discuss more personal psychological strategies which you can apply in everyday life. There is some cross-over or repetition of ideas mentioned in earlier chapters but the significance and overall effectiveness of the following has proven to be so good that they are worth giving more attention to.

TRACING YOUR ILLNESS TO ITS ROOT CAUSE

This can be achieved by completing the following exercise, thus identifying the contributing factors in your life events, possible contributing personality traits which you may want to change in the future. It also addresses your strengths and weaknesses at an emotional level.

Write about the following:

1. The precipitating event, if known – what caused the event? e.g., Death of a partner, spouse, accident/injury, high blood pressure, neglected infections, etc.

2. The belief system – how do you perceive the diagnosis? What are you saying to yourself about the illness, what are your assumptions? Do you accept or deny that you have the illness? Do you feel you can become free of it? How can you change your lifestyle accordingly? Is the illness the signal

button for change? Do you feel time is running out?

3. Consequent emotional reactions – what emotions are disturbed?

(a) Is there resentment against what has happened?

(b) Is there guilt? Do you feel you brought about this illness?

(c) Is there anxiety? Do you feel the need to become dependant on other people? Have you ever had the need to rely on other people for anything in your life?

(d) Perhaps there is a combination of two, or all three of these emotions.

4. Counter-acting questions, e.g., why should the illness demoralise you [e.g., when people become incontinent, patients might need tube feeding, etc.].

A POSITIVE MENTAL ATTITUDE

The importance of positive thinking in recovery from ill health is often undermined in these technology dominated times. However, if asked individually, most people will acknowledge how uplifting a positive outlook can be when people are ill.

As Bernie Siegal says, in his best selling book, *Peace, Love and Healing* 'we kill people by saying a disease is 100% fatal, there is then no hope'. Even those who have been diagnosed with a terminal illness, can find great comfort in optimism. Such optimism can, in some cases, lead to more fulfilled lives even if the final prognosis remains unchanged.

Billings and Moos two English psychologists in the 1980s put forward a very useful list of coping strategies. All of these coping strategies will enhance positive attitudes. Here, we consider some of these attitudes:

1. Try to see the positive aspect of illness – as we discussed already illness can change your life. Treatment is extremely important, and finding the balance between traditional and complementary procedures is in itself a challenge.
2. Try to be objective – otherwise you suffer from what we call the 'why me syndrome?' This makes the sufferer feel very isolated and believe they are alone in suffering from any illness.
3. Prayer/reflection – many individuals find solace in praying/reflection for guidance and strength. Prayer/reflection provide us with the opportunity to take 'time out' and in doing so we can see things much more clearly. Also it helps us to relax the mind.
4. Take things one step at a time – by adopting this approach you avoid the 'what if – syndrome?' e.g., what will happen if I can't take any more medication? What will happen if they refuse to give me chemotherapy? etc.
5. Consider several alternatives for handling the problem – i.e., explore all options and discuss them openly with your doctor. Building up a good rapport with any professional you are dealing with, provides you with a relaxed forum for asking questions to alleviate unnecessary fears.Never try any form of treatment without first discussing it with your doctor. Most doctors now recognise the advantages of complementary techniques and are supportive.
6. Draw on past experiences – ask yourself how you have coped with previous crises in your life. Call on family/friends to point out your positive coping skills .

7. Find out all you can about your illness – talk to other sufferers, read as much as you can, join a support group, even think about starting up a group yourself.

8. Talk to a professional person – do not be afraid to get a second opinion. No doctor or professional will be offended or put out if you ask for a referral for a second opinion.

9. Take some positive action – agree to go for treatment, be patient. Treatment does not always work immediately. Also it is important to note, what works for one patient may not necessarily work for you. There are times when your illness will require some flexibility. Expect this from the outset.

10. Talk with your partner, relatives or friends about the problem in a non-moaning fashion. If you continuously moan, you will find that people will start to visit less and less. Joan Collins in her book *My Secrets* discusses how she ends contact with people who are constantly negative and complaining personalities.

11. Try to keep up a minimum level of exercise – check this with your doctor first. Remember exercise helps to reduce tension. Exercise can be as simple as three, twenty minute walks weekly. Swimming is also recommended for many conditions such as arthritis or back pain.

12. Be prepared for and acknowledge the worst – e.g., treatment may not work initially, or you have been told you only have a short time to live, etc. If you are prepared in this fashion anything positive is an added bonus.

13. Express negative as well as positive emotions – do not hide your fears or your anger. Do not be

afraid to be seen to cry. This does not make you weak or frail. You are being human and you will feel so much better afterwards. One technique that Dr Moore-Groarke uses with her patients is a visualisation technique where she asks them to imagine that their life and feelings are like a well that is gone dry. When a well goes dry it soon fills with algae, dirt, etc. As soon as the tears flow, imagine that water is returning to the well and the difference is enormous.

14. Keep busy – otherwise you surrender and become a victim to your condition. Have an agenda set out for yourself each day. In the agenda include some time for relaxation. You will use your time more efficiently and you will rule your illness rather than your illness ruling you.

SELF-IMAGE AND SELF-ESTEEM

Improving your self-esteem and self-image invariably leads to a better outlook on life and consequently a better approach to your health is adopted. Dr Moore-Groarke encourages patients to fill out the following questionnaire on a regular basis and to try and improve their score, by taking positive steps to communicate better with other people, to practise self-care and to attend to any of their physical, social or emotional needs. The higher the score the greater your self-esteem. It is a useful exercise to compare scores over a given period of time.

Each of the statements below can be rated with the words *Never, Sometimes, Frequently* or *Always*. Make your choice, then write in the number that corresponds to the word you have chosen.

1	2	3	4
Never	Sometimes	Frequently	Always

1. When my feelings are hurt I express this

2. Others value my opinions

3. I feel intellectually capable

4. I feel worthy of the gifts that have been offered to me

5. I am satisfied with my personal development up to now

6. I consider comparing myself with other people to be a waste of time

7. I enjoy meeting and talking with new people

8. I feel comfortable at social gatherings

9. I am happy to be me and wouldn't want to be anyone else

10. I like my present life situation

11. I am happy with the way I live my life

12. I like my present place of residence

13. I enjoy my work

14. People admire me

15. I am considerate of others

16. I enjoy getting up in the morning

17. I am self-reliant

18. I make a positive contribution to the lives
    of others

19. I enjoy attending to my own needs; eating,
    exercise and general care of myself

20. I try to make sure I lead a balanced life – enough
    rest, work play

21. I enjoy my time alone

22. I like myself

23. I respect myself

24. I value myself

25. I see myself as a good-looking person

26. I think of myself as a loving person

27. I think of myself as a sharing person

28. I think of myself as a confident person

29. I see myself as a successful person

TOTAL:_____

Amanda who is 18, had rheumatoid arthritis when she first presented for stress management and time management skills. The first thing her psychologist became aware of was Amanda's poor self-perception. She scored a miserable 46 on the self-esteem questionnaire. Clearly she had to work on how she saw herself and for 6 weeks the focus of her therapy was on improving her self-esteem. When she filled out the questionnaire 6 weeks later her score had doubled (95). She was encouraged to ask those close to her what they felt were her good personality traits. She was amazed that they saw her as reliable, sociable, sharing, loving, etc. She started to believe in herself.

EMOTIONAL MATURITY

Resolving old tensions whether with family or friends releases energy which can free the mind of worry and be utilised by the body to heal itself. Such emotional releases include forgiving others for old hurts as well as forgiving yourself for past faults or mistakes.

Some therapists encourage clients to engage in much forgiveness work with the 'inner child'. In other words, to work through unresolved issues in childhood, e.g., any kind of abuse, domestic violence and to address your feelings as a child, when such occurrences took place. By addressing these feelings you are letting go and forgiving yourself/or sometimes (but not always) the perpetrators of such actions. One of the easiest ways of doing this is by writing a letter to, for example, the perpetrator of the domestic violence, abuse, etc., describing in detail your feeling, your fears and the effect his/her actions had on your life and discussing it and working through it with your therapist. You can then burn the letter.

Staying out of or separating yourself from other people's emotional reactions is also a very useful strategy. Not getting entangled in such emotions can actually preserve energy which can be put to better use. This is where sometimes, an avoidance strategy can be useful. Expressing love to those around you can also nurture positive energy which in turn gets reflected back on yourself.

Being honest with yourself and others about your illness prevents the development of fabrications, half truths and misunderstandings, all of which are a hindrance when someone is clearly fighting to get better. Being honest about help or care that is beneficial allows the sick person to maintain a certain amount of control over their circumstances and a better sense of independence.

By not facing up to how you really feel regarding your illness, often leads you to put on a 'brave face' around your loved ones, especially if you have young children. This puts huge stress on you, and if allowed to continue, can lead to depression. Do not be afraid to talk to your children about your illness. Ask for professional help if you feel you cannot do this yourself. This is usually addressed in counselling, where counselling is available to such patients.

Do not be afraid to express your fears, particularly if you are afraid you are going to die. If you have a terminal illness, preparation for 'death' is important.

BE CREATIVE

You don't have to have a recognised talent to enjoy the creative process. The extra time available during periods of convalescence can provide you with a space to indulge yourself in a pleasurable pastime whether it be playing a musical instrument, planting a garden, painting, cooking, writing, sewing, etc. Using your imagination in this way sometimes opens the mind to a fuller experience of illness which can in itself lead to a brighter road to recovery (Audrey's case history in Chapter 5 exemplifies this).

Several people have written books on their experiences of illness, in an attempt to encourage others to face the road to recovery a little easier.

LEAVE TIME FOR YOUR SPIRIT

Whether you find your spirit in a church, up a mountain, on a park bench or in your garden, illness can present an opportunity which releases you from a busy schedule to free your mind, quieten your emotions and let your spirit free. Calm reflection comes in different ways to different people but it rarely leaves without giving some insight into yourself as well as a better understanding of your relationships with others. Listening to this inner voice can provide some helpful thoughts on how to deal with the future.

During illness people often recognise feelings of guilt, for the first time in years, if you have 'unfinished business' with a family member or friend. The need to become reconciled with such individuals can become a priority. Often a sense of relief, calmness and inner-peace follows if such actions are taken. In this way illness can help us lead a better life with more caring and forgiving attitudes. Bitterness regarding an illness and to others because of the illness does nothing to aid recovery, if anything it retards it. You may not necessarily get rid of these negative feelings but at least you can attempt to free your mind (if you find these feelings are beginning to consume you) through therapy and/or relaxation.

IMPROVE THE QUALITY OF YOUR LIFE

Since the 1980s much research has been carried out on quality of life. Quality of life is measured under the following headings:

(a) Physical activity – e.g., work, study, managing ones household.
(b) Daily living – e.g., eating, washing, toileting, dressing, using public or private transport.

(c) Health – physical well-being and stamina.
(d) Support – from relatives or friends.
(e) Outlook – appearing calm and positive, being troubled, confused, frightened, etc.

If any of these areas of our lives change, they put a huge strain on us emotionally. As an exercise make a list of any changes that have occurred in any of these areas of your life. Discuss them with your doctor or psychologist and discover new ways of coping.

By completing some or all of these exercises, you have the basis of many therapy sessions, and are well on the path of creating a better way. As Max Erhmann in 'Desiderata' says: 'But do not distress yourself with imaginings. Many fears are born of fatigue and loneliness. Beyond a wholesome discipline, be gentle with yourself'.

Useful Addresses

The following is a list of some of the places where help/treatment is available. It is advisable first of all to contact your GP who may be able to put you in touch with a local professional or some source of help in your area.

Psychological and Counselling Services
Dr Gillian Moore-Groarke,
Consultant Psychologist,
Suite 21,
Cork Clinic,
Western Road,
Cork.
Tel: (021) 343073

St Francis Medical Centre,
Ballinderry,
Mullingar,
Co. Westmeath.
Tel: (044) 51500

Clanwilliam Institute:
18 Clanwilliam Terrace,
Grand Canal Quay,
Dublin 2.
Tel: (01) 6761363

Directory of registered psychologists:
Psychological Society of Ireland,
13 Adelaide Road,
Dublin 2.
Tel: (01) 4783916

Directory of Chartered Psychologists:
British Psychological Society,
St Andrews House,
48 Princes Rd.,
East Leicester LE1 7DR,
U.K.
Tel: 0116 254 9568

Directory of Accredited Counsellors:
Irish Association of Counselling,
9 Tivoli Terrace,
Dun Laoghaire East,
Dublin.
Tel: (01) 2844752

British Association for Counselling:
1 Regent Place,
Rugby,
Warwickshire CV21 2PJ,
U.K.
Tel: 0788 550899

Neurological Clinics
Cork University Hospital,
Wilton,
Cork.
Tel: (021) 546400

Limerick Regional Hospital,
Dooradoyle,
Limerick.
Tel. (061) 301111

Adelaide Hospital,
Peter Street,
Dublin 8.
Tel: (01) 4758971

St Vincent's Hospital,
Elm Park,
Dublin 4.
Tel: (01) 2694533

University Hospital,
Galway.
Tel: (091) 24222

*N.B. In Ireland patients must obtain a covering letter from their doc-
tor before requesting an appointment for consultation, in any of
the above clinics.*

Physical Disease Societies
Irish Cancer Society,
5 Northumberland Road,
Dublin 4. Tel: (01) 6681855*
They will provide you with details of your local support
group.
Free Phone Cancer Helpline: 1800 200 300 (9 am–5 pm, Monday
to Friday)

Irish Heart Foundation,
4 Clyde Road,
Ballsbridge,
Dublin 4.
Tel: (01) 6685001

Arthritis Foundation,
1 Clanwilliam Square,
Grand Canal Quay,
Dublin 2.
Tel: (01) 6618188

Asthma Society of Ireland,
15 Eden Quay,
Dublin 1.
Tel: (01) 8788511
Asthma Information Line: 1850 445464 (Thursday afternoons)

Irish Society of Crohn's Disease and Colitis,
Carmichael House,
North Brunswick Street,
Dublin 7.
Tel: (01) 8721416

Mental, Physical and Spiritual Healing Addresses
The Irish Hospice Foundation,
64 Waterloo Road,
Dublin 4.
Tel: (01) 6603111

Crystalis,
Donard,
Co. Wicklow. Tel: (045) 54713
They run weekend programmes which explore spirituality.

Creative Counselling Centre,
7 Park Road,
Dun Laoghaire,
Co. Dublin.
Tel: (01) 2841169

The Society of Teachers of the Alexander Technique,
10 London House,
266 Fulham Road,
London SW10 GEL,
England.

Slanú,
Holy Trinity Convent,
Ballyloughaun Rd.,
Renmore,
Galway. Tel: (091) 55023
Contact: Maureen Murphy
Help centre adopting a holistic approach for cancer patients.

Aware,
Helping to Beat Depression,
147 Phibsboro Rd.,
Dublin 7.
Tel: (01) 6791711 (Helpline)
Tel: (01) 8308449 (Administration)

Bereavement Counselling,
Sernie,
St Anne's Church,
Dawson Street,
Dublin 2. Tel: (01) 6767727
Mon. & Wed.: 7.45–9.45pm.

Miscellaneous Addresses
Irish Yoga Association,
108 Lower Kimmage Rd.,
Harold's Cross,
Dublin 6W.
Tel: (01) 281990

T'ai Chi Association of Ireland,
St Andrews Resource Centre,
114 Pearse St.,
Dublin 2.
Tel: (01) 6771930

Aikedo Association of Ireland,
26 Pearse St.,
Dublin 2.
Tel: (01) 6718454

British Migraine Association,
178 A High Rd.,
Byfleet,
Weybridge,
Surrey KT 147 ED.,
U.K.
Tel: 0044 1932 352 468

International Association for the Study of Pain,
Westland Building, Room 301,
1309 Summit Avenue,
Seattle, W.A. 98101.
Tel: 001 206 547 6409

Health Promotion Unit,
Hawkins House,
Dublin 2.
Tel: (01) 6714711

Irish Society of Chartered Physiotherapists,
Royal College of Surgeons,
St Stephen's Green,
Dublin 2.
Tel: (01) 4780200

Eating disorder Assoc.
Sackville Place,
44–48 Magdelen Street,
Norwich,
Norfolk NR3 1JE.
Tel: 01603 621 414

Irish Patient's Association,
78 Seafield Court,
Killiney,
Co. Dublin.

N.B. Some services will be covered by your local health board, or you may be able to claim benefit from private medical insurance schemes. Many therapists operate a sliding scale fee system, so do not be afraid to ask. It is your responsibility to check the credentials of the therapist.

The above list is published for information purposes only. As not every form of treatment is suitable for all people it would be prudent and advisable to consult with a general practitioner before embarking on any course of treatment. Dr Moore-Groarke will not accept patient referrals without a general practitioner's letter.

BIBLIOGRAPHY

Bakal, Donald A., *Psychology and Medicine, Psychobiological Dimensions of Health and Sickness*. Tavistock Publications, London 1979.

Beliauskas, Lias A., *Stress and its Relationship to Health and Illness*. Westview Press, UK 1982.

Billings, A. G., and Moos, R. H., 'The role of coping responses in athenuating the stress of life events', *J. Beh. Med.*, 4 (2), pp. 139–157, 1981.

Chopra, Deepak, *Quantum Healing – Exploring the Frontiers of Mind/ Body Medicine*. Bantam Books, NY 1990.

Cousins, Norman, *Anatomy of an Illness*. Bantam Books, NY 1987.

Davis, Martha, Eshelman, Eliz, Mc Kay, Mathew, *The relaxation and stress reduction workbook*. New Harbinger Publications, CA 1988.

Gawler, Ian, *You can conquer cancer*. Thorsons, UK 1986.

Hay, Louise, L., *You Can Heal Your Life*. Eden Grove edition, UK 1988.

Hoffmanm, David, *The Holistic Herbal Way to Successful Stress Control*. Thorsons, UK 1986.

Illich, Ivan, *Limits to Medicine*. Penguin, UK 1977.

Kobasa, S. C., 'The Hardy Personality – Towards a Social Psychology of Stress and Health', in Sanders G. S., Suls, J. [eds], *Social Psychology of Health and Illness*. Lawrence Erlbaum, Hillsdale, NJ 1982.

Lipton, Sampson, *Conquering Pain*. Positive Health Guide, Martin Dunitz Ltd, London 1984.

Mathews, A., Steptoe, A., *Essential Psychology for Medical Practice*. Churchill Livingstone, Longman Group, UK 1988.

McCarthy, Margot, *Natural Therapies – The Complete A-Z of Complementary Health*. Thorsons, UK 1995.

Melzack, R., 'The McGill Pain Questionnaire: major properties and scoring methods', *Pain*, 1, pp. 277–299, 1975.

Moore-Groarke, Gillian, Thompson, Sylvia, *When food becomes your enemy.* Mercier Press, Cork/Dublin 1995.

Moore-Groarke, Gillian, *Relaxation tape for overcoming stress.* Sulan Studios, Cork 1992.

Ornstein, Robert and Sobel, David, *The Healing Brain.* Macmillan, UK 1988.

Robins, Trevor R., Cooper Peter, J., *Psychology for Medicine.* Edward Arnold, UK 1988.

Russell, Michael L., *Stress Management for Chronic Disease.* Pergamon General Psychology series, UK 1988.

Siegal, Bernie, *Peace, Love and Healing – Body Mind Communication and the Path to Self-Healing.* Rider, UK 1990.

Simonton, O. C., Matthews-Simonton, S. and Creighton, J. L., *Getting well again.* Bantam Books, New York, 1980.

Simonton, Stephanie, M., *The Healing Family – the Simonton Approach for Families facing Illness.* Bantam Books, New York 1988.

Stanway, Andrew, *Alternative Medicine – A guide to Natural Therapies.* Penguin Books, UK 1982.

Totman, Richard, *Mind, Stress and Health.* Souvenir Press, UK 1990.

Tuck, Denis C., *Health, Illness and Families, a lifespan perspective.* Wiley Press, New York 1985.

Wasserman, Havey, *The Healing Road.* Auburn House, Ireland 1995.

Wilber Ken, *Grace & Grit.* Gill & Macmillian, Dublin 1991.

Wilkonson, Marcia, *Migraine and Headaches – Understanding, Controlling and Avoiding the Pain.* Positive Health Guide, Martin Dunitz Ltd, London1982.